# PERINATAL DEPRESSION

Edited by **María Graciela Rojas Castillo**

**Perinatal Depression**
Edited by María Graciela Rojas Castillo

**Published by InTech**

Janeza Trdine 9, 51000 Rijeka, Croatia



**Publishing Process Manager** Oliver Kurelic

**Technical Editor** Teodora Smiljanic

**Cover Designe**r InTech Design Team

Additional hard copies can be obtained from orders@intechopen.com

Perinatal Depression, Edited by María Graciela Rojas Castillo
p. cm.
ISBN 978-953-307-826-7

For EU product safety concerns:
IN TECH d.o.o., Prolaz Marije Krucifikse Kozulić 3, 51000 Rijeka, Croatia,
info@intechopen.com or visit our website at intechopen.com.

# Meet the editor

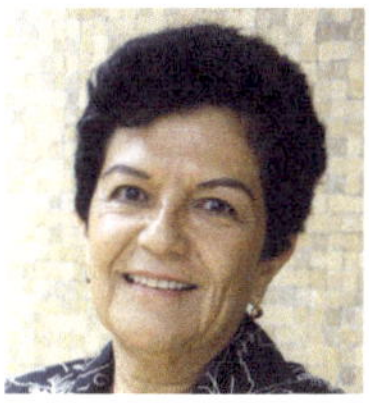

Graciela Rojas, MD, is a Professor of Psychiatry at the Faculty of Medicine of the University of Chile, Santiago. She is also the Deputy Director and prior to that was the Director of the Psychiatric Clinic at the University of Chile for eight years. She has been working in different research projects for 20 years and has participated in a series of intervention trials to improve the treatment of depression in primary care in her country. In 2002 she has been awarded a large grant to carry out the first randomized clinical trial of the treatment of postnatal depression in Latin America. Now she is a Principal Investigator in a randomized clinical trial with the objective to compare the effectiveness of a telemedicine-based collaborative program with usual care in rural primary care clinics. She participated in the Regional Network for Mental Health Research in Latin America funded by the NIMH, and is also member of several important Training committees such as the Doctor of Public Health Program.

# Contents

# Preface

Depression is a common mental disorder throughout the world. It is more frequent among women and in developing countries.

Parenthood is a very important role in life of a person and represents many challenges for individuals and for the society.

Depression can be suffered during pregnancy and in the postpartum period. Postpartum depression is a common subtype of depression that can have negative effects on the mother, the infant and the family.

Understanding the biological, psychological and social basis of perinatal depression is very important for the design of treatment programs, and so far several psychological and pharmacological treatments have been successfully used to treat depression.

However, even when the evidence shows that depression can be treated, it remains sub-detected and sub-treated with deleterious effects for the population.

With this book we want to contribute to better understanding of perinatal anxiety and depression, their impact on mother-child relationship and better detection of the depression among mothers.

We also wanted to remark that men, as well, can be depressed in the postpartum period.

Minorities, immigrants and the rural population were also considered with three different chapters.

**María Graciela Rojas Castillo**
Clinical Hospital, Faculty of Medicine, University of Chile, Santiago, Chile

# 1

# Screening and Prevention of Postnatal Depression

Kari Glavin
*Diakonova University College, Oslo, Norway*

## 1. Introduction

Pregnancy and the period following delivery represent a major transition in life with changes and challenges. The distinction between a natural response to this transition and a disorder requiring treatment can be difficult to detect, both for a new mother and for people in her surroundings. For many women, this is a period of increased psychological vulnerability and distress, which is detectable across a broad spectrum of reactions with consequences for the woman's well-being, for bonding between the mother and child, and for the whole family (Cox & Holden, 2003; Kendall-Tackett, 2005).

The literature commonly describes three types of distress: postnatal blues, postnatal depression, and postnatal psychosis. Postnatal blues (mood instability and mild depression) is a relatively normal reaction to a central experience in life that can be regarded as a release of tension after a birth. It is experienced by 50–80% of all women. This is a passing emotional instability during the first days after birth. Sleep problems, concentration problems, crying easily and reduced appetite are common signs of postnatal blues (Kendall-Tackett, 2005; Wheatley, 2005). This reaction is normal and needs only information to the parents as well as understanding from staff at the maternity ward (Wheatley, 2005). It is a warning sign if this condition does not disappear within a short time; an extended period of blues may be a sign of emerging postnatal depression. As the stay in the maternity ward after birth is often very short, health practitioners in primary care play an important role in recognizing a possibly severe and prolonged 'blues' reaction (Wickberg & Hwang, 2003).

The most serious form of psychological reaction after birth is postnatal psychosis, which occurs in about one or two per 1000 births (Brockington, 2004a; O'Hara, 1987; Wickberg & Hwang, 2003). This is an acute psychotic reaction, normally occurring soon after the first week following birth (Brockington, 2004a; Wickberg & Hwang, 2003). Postnatal psychosis has high and specific heritability. The risk of postnatal psychosis is higher for women who have bipolar disorder (Brockington, 2004a). Warning signs of birth psychosis are deep depression, mania, obsessions and disorientation. The condition needs special treatment, but the prognosis is good if the condition is detected in time (Brockington, 2004a; Wickberg & Hwang, 2003).

Postnatal depression is the focus of this chapter. Prevalence studies of postnatal depression have used different screening tools and different points of time for screening. The prevalence of postnatal depression in these studies ranges from zero to almost 60% (Halbreich & Karkun, 2006). In some countries, there are few reports of postnatal depression, whereas in other countries reported postpartum depressive symptoms are very prevalent. It is well documented that postnatal depression affects at least 10% of all mothers within the first postpartum year (Cox & Holden, 2003; Gordon et al., 2006; Halbreich & Karkun, 2006; Kendall-Tackett, 2005).

The term 'postnatal depression' is useful to describe any depressive disorder without psychotic features present within the first year following childbirth (Cox & Holden, 2003). An indication of postnatal depression is a low mood that causes every day to be experienced as heavy and grey. Forgetfulness, concentration problems, reduced self-esteem and feelings of failing as a mother are the dominant symptoms. Other common reactions are sleeping problems, appetite loss, extreme tiredness, anxiety, guilt, loss of energy, and indecisiveness. Some women experience loss of control over their existence, which can lead to an increasing feeling of unease, irritability and outbreaks of anger, inability to cope, and thoughts of suicide (Cox &Holden, 2003; Dennis & Creedy, 2004; Kendall-Tackett, 2005; Wickberg & Hwang, 2003). Depression ranges in severity from mild, temporary episodes of sadness to severe, persistent depression. The term "clinical depression" is used to describe the more severe, persistent form of depression also known as "major depression" or "major depressive disorder" (Snoek & Engedal, 2000). As regards the symptoms or frequency of occurrence, postnatal depression does not differ from depressions in other life periods (Brockington, 2004a; Cooper & Murray, 1998; O'Hara et al., 1990; Wickberg & Hwang, 2003).

However, a mother's depression may affect her relationship with her child, as well as the quality of care she provides. Due to disturbed maternal sensitivity, the child may develop an insecure attachment to its mother, which may affect the child's later emotional and cognitive development (Campbell et al., 2004; Dennis, 2004; McLearn et al., 2006). Maternal depressive symptoms might also contribute to unfavourable parenting practices (McLearn et al., 2006), and depressed mothers report higher parenting stress than non-depressed mothers (Abidin, 1995; Glavin et al., 2010b; Morrell et al., 2009a). Early intervention through primary health services within the existing system has been shown to prevent long-term postnatal depression (Brugha et al., 2011; Dennis & Creedy, 2004; Elliott et al., 2001; Glavin et al., 2009, 2010b). Thus, identifying and treating postnatal depression as early as possible may be essential. The aim of this chapter is to describe identification of postnatal depression, various screening instruments, appropriate points of time for screening, follow-up of screening, and potential for prevention of postnatal depression.

## 2. Identification of postnatal depression

In spite of growing evidence that postnatal depression can be effectively treated and possibly prevented (Brugha et al., 2011; Glavin et al., 2010a, 2010b; Morrell et al., 2009a), this disturbance is still undetected or untreated in many women (Dennis, 2009). Several barriers to detection and treatment are described: women lack knowledge about postnatal depression, they deny or minimize their symptoms, they assume their problems are common after giving birth, or they are not aware of the treatment options. Barriers among clinicians and in the healthcare system, as well as economic and personal factors, caused low treatment rates among a sample of at-risk women (Horowitz & Cousins, 2006). Health professionals can trivialize the symptoms or offer treatment that is not suitable for the women (Dennis, 2009; Dennis & Chung-Lee, 2006).

As many women do not report physical or emotional disorders after childbirth, the primary health care service does not adequately address these women's needs (Cox & Holden, 2003; MacArthur et al., 2003). Universal screening for postnatal depression during well-child care visits has been shown to increase detection (Morrell et al., 2009a; McLearn et al., 2006; Glavin et al., 2010c). There is a need for comprehensive screening programmes and better organization of care for preventing and treating postnatal depression (Dennis, 2009). According to McLearn et al. (2006), identification, guidance and referral related to women's mental health are a professional responsibility. However, according to Cox & Holden (2003), there is a need for training for all health professionals in managing postnatal depression. The training should include the nature, detection and treatment of postnatal depression. Recent studies provide evidence that health professionals can be trained to identify, prevent and treat postnatal depression in women (Brugha et al., 2011; Glavin et al., 2010a, 2010b, 2010c; Morrell et al., 2009a, 2009b). Nurses are well positioned to counsel depressed mothers about treatment options, to make recommendations and to provide referrals (Horowitz & Goodman, 2005; Wickberg & Hwang, 2003; Glavin et al., 2010b).

Brockington (2004b) states that the merit of a broad concept of postnatal depression is the public recognition that postpartum disorders are common, promoting the development of remedial services. The use of clinical criteria and diagnosis is independent of when the diseases arise. The International Classification of Diseases (ICD-10) recommends that depression in the postpartum period is categorized in one of the established categories (WHO, 1992), whereas the Diagnostic and Statistical Manual of Mental Disorder revision IV (DSM-IV) accepts an extra coding that specifies when the disease arose (American Psychiatric Association, 1994). According to Cox (2004), however, these diagnostic manuals are not well suited for use in the postpartum period as the ICD-10 permits the classification of mental and behavioural disorders associated with the puerperium only if they onset within six weeks and if they cannot be classified elsewhere, and the DSM-IV with an even shorter onset of four weeks.

### 2.1 Screening instruments

A valid method of screening for postnatal depression implies that health care workers have a tool available to help them in identifying women with thoughts related to postnatal depression. Health practitioners such as public health nurses (PHNs), midwives and nurses have an important task in identifying and treating women with postnatal depression. The aim is early establishment of offers of help, and referrals when necessary. The development of screening instruments gives the primary health services an opportunity for early identification of postnatal depression. Many studies have shown that screening can increase detection rates (Georgiopoulos et al., 2001; Glavin et al., 2010c; Wickberg & Hwang, 2003). In a study by Georgiopoulos et al. (2001), the rate of postnatal depression diagnosis increased from 3.7% before the routine use of EPDS screening to 10.7% when universal screening with EPDS was implemented.

Questionnaires in common use are the General Health Questionnaire (GHQ), the Beck Depression Inventory (BDI), the Postpartum Depression Screening Scale (PDSS) and the

Edinburgh Postnatal Depression Scale (EPDS) (Brockington, 2004a; Cox et al., 1987; Cox & Holden, 2003). In a recent review by Zubaran et al. (2010), four screening tools were reviewed and compared. The Edinburgh Postnatal Depression Scale (EPDS) and the Postpartum Depression Screening Scale (PDSS) showed substantial sensitivity and specificity as screening tools. However, when applied to different cultural contexts, none of the instruments could be rated as flawless. The most commonly used screening tool for postnatal depression is the EPDS (Fitelson et al., 2010). In this chapter, the focus will be on the EPDS as a screening instrument for the primary health care service.

### 2.1.1 The General Health Questionnaire (GHQ)

The GHQ has been developed as a screening tool to detect those likely to have or to be at risk of developing psychiatric disorders, and is available in a variety of versions using 12, 28, 30 or 60 items; the 28-item version is used most widely (Jackson, 2007).

### 2.1.2 Beck's Depression Inventory (BDI)

The BDI is a 21-question multiple-choice self-report inventory, and is an instrument for measuring the severity of depression (Lee et al., 2000; Kendall-Tackett, 2005).

### 2.1.3 The Postpartum Depression Screening Scale (PDSS)

Like the EPDS, and in contrast to the GHQ and the BDI, the PDSS is a screening tool designed specifically for new mothers, and is a 35-item self-report instrument (Kendall-Tackett, 2005). The PDSS is considered effective for identifying minor and major depression (Zubaran et al., 2010). Studies have demonstrated the reliability, construct validity, and sound psychometric properties of the PDSS (Beck & Gable, 2000; Zubaran et al., 2010). PDSS-SF is the short version of PDSS and consists of seven items. According to Zubaran et al. (2010), the PDSS-SF is useful as it provides a "quick, but accurate, overall level of postpartum depression symptomatology".

### 2.1.4 The Edinburgh Postnatal Depression Scale

Cox et al. (1987) developed this 10-item self-report instrument to detect depressive symptoms among women who have just given birth. The questionnaire has been translated into several languages. The EPDS was developed and validated against the Research Diagnostic Criteria for depression to identify and screen for depression postpartum (Cox, 2004). It is a general screening tool for the whole range of postpartum psychiatric disorders. A positive score needs to be followed by an interview clarifying the symptoms of depression (Brockington, 2004b; Cox & Holden, 2003). The EPDS focuses on the cognitive and affective features of depression rather than somatic symptoms. The scale alone can not confirm a diagnosis of depression, but it is widely used to indicate probable depressive disorder. The EPDS does not screen for those at risk for becoming depressed in the future, but it will identify mild depression and prevent a severe prolonged disorder (Cox & Holden, 2003).

The screening form consists of ten questions, each offering four response alternatives. It takes about five minutes to complete the form. The EPDS is easy to score; each item is rated on a 4-point scale (from 0 to 3), yielding a summary score of 0-30. A higher score indicates more severe symptoms. A score of 0-9 indicates no risk of experiencing symptoms of postnatal depression; a score of 10-12 indicates a minor/major risk of experiencing symptoms of postnatal depression; and a score of 13 or greater indicates a major risk of experiencing symptoms of postnatal depression (Cox & Holden, 2003; Lanes et al., 2011). Independently of the score, a special note should be made of any positive responses to item 10 assessing suicidal ideation. A positive score on item 10 should be taken seriously and action taken (Cox & Holden, 2003).

The scale assesses the intensity of depressive symptoms present within the previous seven days. The instrument has been used both in clinical settings and in epidemiological studies, and is generally well accepted by women (Cox et al. 1996; Segre et al., 2010). Even if variability in sensitivity and specificity occurs across languages and cultures, the sensitivity and specificity of the EPDS has been found to be satisfactory in several studies (Cox & Holden, 2003; Berle et al., 2003; Wickberg & Hwang, 2003; Lanes et al., 2011). The instrument is described as a valid, reliable and economical screening tool (Buist et al., 2002), and has been recommended for postpartum screening (Georgiopoulos et al., 2001; Wickberg & Hwang, 2003).

According to Glavin et al. (2010c), public health nurses regarded the EPDS as very valuable, and they were convinced that they had identified more mothers with postnatal depression than they had done previously. Georgiopoulos et al. (2001) also found that EPDS screening at 6 weeks postpartum increased the rate of diagnosed postnatal depression. The public health nurses in the study by Glavin et al. (2010c) described the EPDS as being easy for the mothers to complete and for the nurses to score. Other studies using the EPDS as a screening instrument postpartum also found that EPDS is simple and easy to use for health care workers and mothers (Freeman et al., 2005; Georgiopoulos et al., 1999; Seeley et al., 1996).

Krantz et al. (2008) argued that routine EPDS screening of postpartum women would lead to considerable ethical problems due to the weak scientific foundation of the screening instrument. They argue that the side effects in terms of misclassifications have not been considered carefully and that the EPDS does not function well as a routine screening instrument. However, the public health nurses in the study by Glavin et al. (2010c) perceived the EPDS as a suitable, well accepted and useful screening tool that led to better identification of women with postnatal depression than had been the case previously. Other researchers also report that EPDS is well accepted by women, and health staff confirm that they identify more women with postnatal depression using the tool (Mason & Poole, 2008; Vik et al., 2009). According to Buist et al. (2002), there is also a concern that women who yield a "false positive" result may become anxious after the screening. The public health nurses in the study by Glavin et al. (2010c) did not report such problems. The reason may be the feedback the women received following completion of the EPDS at 6 weeks postpartum. The public health nurses talked with the mother about her mental health and her feelings after she had completed the EPDS. The author of the EPDS (Cox & Holden, 2003) and the guidelines for its use (Coyle & Adams, 2002) confirm the importance of this feedback to the mother. According to Glavin et al. (2010c), the EPDS increased the focus on postnatal depression, and it functioned as a door opener for the public health nurses. Other studies also show that the EPDS can be used as a starting point for conversations about the mother's psychological condition (Buist et al., 2002; Cooper & Murray, 1998; Cox et al., 1987). Public health nurses reported that the parents provided positive reports about the screening procedure (Glavin et al., 2010c). Several studies support the acceptability of the EPDS for mothers when it is used appropriately (Freeman et al., 2005; Georgiopoulos et al., 1999; Milgrom et al., 2005; Poole et al., 2006; Segre et al., 2010).

A question raised in the literature is whether the EPDS measures only depression, or both depression and anxiety. In a validation study by Vivilaki et al. (2009), a factor analysis confirmed the multidimensionality of the EPDS, demonstrating a two-factor structure that contained subscales reflecting depressive symptoms and anxiety. In another study, Montazeri et al. (2007) also found that the EPDS not only measures postnatal depression but may also be measuring anxiety. Navarro et al. (2007) concluded that the EPDS is a valid instrument to detect postnatal depression as well as postnatal anxiety and adjustment disorders; thus, it has to be considered whether the instrument measures more than depression. According to Montazeri et al. (2007), one may argue that the EPDS is a general measure of psychological distress rather than a one-dimensional measure of depression. Brockington (2004b) states that the trinity classification of maternity blues, postpartum depression and postnatal psychosis is an oversimplification. He states that the concept of postpartum depression is broad and that mothers with postpartum depression constitute a heterogeneous group with a broad spectrum of postpartum psychiatric disorders. According to Brockington (2004b), a four-part classification may be more appropriate: psychoses, mother-infant relationship disorders, depression, and a miscellaneous group of anxiety and stress-related disorders. Brockington (2004b) is of the opinion that postnatal anxiety disorders may be more common than depression and that they represent an underemphasized entity. The EPDS is widely used for screening of postnatal depression and is judged valuable (Chabrol et al., 2002; Georgiopoulos et al., 2001; Wickberg & Hwang, 2003). However, several researchers argue that the EPDS captures elements of both anxiety and depression (Montazeri et al., 2007; Navarro et al., 2007; Vivilaki et al., 2009). According to Montazeri et al. (2007), this could be regarded as a strength of the EPDS, and an assessment of both anxiety and depression should be done both in the antenatal and postpartum periods. In the study by Glavin et al. (2010b), the increased focus on maternal mental health and supportive counselling sessions yielded a significant decrease in the depression score between the municipalities, and the public health nurses seemed to have prevented and treated cases of postnatal depression. However, it is possible that some of the high scores on the EPDS were caused by anxiety disorders and that the supportive counselling sessions were helpful for anxious women as well. Irrespective of the classification and name of the disorder, it is important to help the women suffering from a postpartum psychiatric disorder and to be aware of both postnatal depression and other possible disorders such as anxiety and stress-related disorders, as mentioned by Brockington (2004b). In any case, the EPDS seems to be a helpful tool to identify women in need of help. Further research is needed on comorbid disorders in the postpartum period, and the possibility to identify and help women suffering from all these conditions.

The EPDS is a screening device and not a diagnostic tool; use of the instrument requires a clinical assessment and a counselling session by a health care worker after the completion of the EPDS (Cox & Holden, 2003). According to Seeley (2001), the EPDS is only as good as the person using it. Depression screening must also be combined with systemic paths for referral of cases and well-defined implemented care plans to achieve outcome benefits (Cox & Holden, 2003; Stewart et al., 2004).

## 2.2 Time for screening

The risk of developing postnatal depression is greatest in the first three months postpartum, decreasing slightly in the fourth through the seventh month after delivery (Beck, 2006). Some residual depressive symptoms are common up to a year after delivery (Beck, 2006; Dennis & Creedy, 2004). Though most of these depressions are of a milder type that disappears after a few months, there is a risk that women will have a longer-term and more difficult depression if they do not receive help. It is therefore important not to trivialize signs of postnatal depression, but to discover the situation early and give the women help and follow-up (Wickberg & Hwang, 2003). Screening for postnatal depression is recommended 6–8 weeks after delivery (Cox & Holden, 2003). Good results have been reported with the use of a screening instrument 6 weeks postpartum (Glavin et al., 2009, 2010b; Morrell et al., 2009a).

## 2.3 Follow-up

New cases of postnatal depression have been found during the whole first year after delivery. In a study by Glavin et al. (2010b), the prevalence rate was 14.4% at 6 weeks, 10.4% at 3 months, 8.8% at 6 months and 5.6% at 12 months, which indicates that health practitioners need to be aware of postnatal depression among women during the whole first postpartum year. Davies et al. (2003) found new cases of depression at 3, 6 and 12 months postpartum and recommended that health visitors should screen for postnatal depression for a longer period, not only in the immediate postpartum period. In a Swedish study, Rubertsson et al. (2005) also found new cases up to 12 months postpartum and recommended strategies to evaluate maternal emotional wellbeing during the entire postpartum period. Postnatal depression often goes undiagnosed and untreated even in women who have had multiple visits to healthcare providers (Driscoll, 2006). These studies suggest that it is important to be aware of new cases and continue to use a screening tool on indication later in the postpartum period in order to prevent and treat new cases of depression.

## 2.4 Implementing a screening procedure

The introduction of a screening instrument entails requirements that are important to take into account. The disease, the screening test and referral system are some of these. The disease should represent an important health problem, appear reasonably often, have a known pattern, and have a latent (asymptomatic) stage of a certain duration, so that early discovery and treatment have a positive influence upon ending the disease (Holland et al., 2006). It is still presupposed that not all of these requirements need to be fulfilled. For postnatal depression, many of these requirements are satisfied; it represents an important health problem that affects the mother, child and family. It appears fairly regularly: 8–15 % of all women who have given birth develop postnatal depression (Buist et al., 2002; Gale & Harlow, 2003; Glavin et al., 2009; Wickberg & Hwang, 2003). Early diagnosis and treatment have a positive effect on the trajectory of the disease (Chabrol et al., 2002; Dennis, 2003; Glavin et al., 2010b; Morrell et al., 2009a; Ray & Hodnett, 2004).

The requirements for a screening test are that it should be simple, acceptable, valid and economical in relation to the results (Holland et al., 2006). The EPDS is a simple test that is easy to administer to all newly fledged mothers. The test has been validated in several countries and its sensitivity and specificity were satisfactory (Berle et al., 2003; Cox & Holden 2003; Wickberg & Hwang, 2003). Sensitivity and specificity are somehow different depending on how high the score for depression is set. However, studies confirm that the EPDS is a valid clinical screening instrument to diagnose postnatal depression (Berle et al., 2003; Cox & Holden, 2003; Wickberg & Hwang, 2003). It should be emphasized that all instruments are screening tools that will generate a certain number of false positives, and a diagnosis of depression must always be confirmed by clinical interview (Fitelson et al., 2010).

## 3. Preventing postnatal depression

Transition to motherhood involves a period of increased psychological vulnerability, and for some women it may be complicated and cause a great deal of stress (Brockington, 2004b; Chick & Meleis, 1986; Kendall-Tackett, 2005). One response to the transition to parenthood may be depression (Chick & Meleis, 1986). Preventing postnatal depression ought to be started during the pregnancy.

### 3.1 Pregnancy

Dreams and plans are important components for mothers who are in the transition to motherhood (Stern & Bruschweiler-Stern, 2000). The mother's mental well-being in pregnancy is of importance for the mother's bonding to the unborn child and for the child after birth (Brodén, 2004). Depression affects approximately 10% of all women during pregnancy (O'Hara, 1986). According to Evans et al. (2001), symptoms of depression are not more common or severe after childbirth than during pregnancy. In a Swedish sample, 37% of the women who had scores above the threshold for probable depression in pregnancy also had a high score postpartum (Rubertsson et al., 2005).

Postnatal depression can develop in primiparous and multiparous women. Risk factors are a previous history of depression, either during pregnancy or at other times, postnatal depression following a previous pregnancy, stressful events during the past year, including illness, job loss or pregnancy complications, marital conflict, a weak support system, and unplanned or unwanted pregnancy (Beck, 2006; Brockington, 2004a; Dennis et al., 2004; Kendall-Tackett, 2005; O'Hara & Swain, 1996). Lanes et al. (2011) found an association between total household income and postpartum depressive symptoms, which were found to decrease as household income increased. Other factors positively associated with postpartum depressive symptoms were immigration status, delivery at a young age, and a prior diagnosis of depression. In this study, the highest direct association with postpartum depressive symptoms was the amount of stress during pregnancy and the lack of availability of support postpartum (Lanes et al., 2011).

According to Beck (2006), there is insufficient evidence that interventions in the pregnancy may prevent postnatal depression. However, in spite of limited evidence, it may be important to inform women about possible mental health problems in the postpartum period, as information to women postpartum has been shown to prevent cases of depressive symptoms among women (Brugha et al., 2011; Glavin et al., 2009, 2010 b, 2010c; Heh & Fu,

2003). Prenatal visits provide an opportunity to inform the parents about possible postpartum mental health disorders and obtain information about a mother's risk factors.

### 3.2 Early discharge from hospital after delivery

According to Brown et al. (2002), early discharge from hospital after delivery may have negative consequences for mothers and babies because decreased maternal confidence is common, due to lack of professional support and higher prevalence of postpartum depression. In a preventive programme, it is important to strengthen the resources of the municipalities to provide support to newly fledged mothers' early discharge from the hospital. More emotional and informational support to parents both in pregnancy and during the postpartum period has been a recommendation made in studies (Deave et al., 2008; Wilkins, 2006), and should be considered important to the primary health care services. Information given to parents during the hospital stay describing mental health conditions that can occur post partum may prevent cases of postnatal depression. In a study by Ho et al. (2009), women who received information about postnatal depression, and an educational programme at the hospital 2 days postpartum experienced less depression 3 months postpartum than the control group.

### 3.3 Peer support

In a randomized controlled trial, Dennis et al. (2009) evaluated the effectiveness of telephone-based peer support on prevention of postnatal depression. They conclude that telephone-based peer support can be effective in preventing postnatal depression among woman at high risk. The women who received peer support had half the risk of developing postnatal depression at 12 weeks postpartum than those in the control group. For some women, there is a need for information and support from others than the nearest family (Brown et al., 2002) and peer support can be an alternative.

### 3.4 Emotional and informational support to parents

Research from the US shows that regular home visits by public health nurses to the family during the child's first two years contribute to preventing emotional, language and mental health problems of children (Olds et al., 2002) as well as child abuse and neglect (Olds et al., 1997). There is also evidence from the UK that home visiting and the detection and management of postnatal depression can produce positive effects on parenting and mother-child interaction (Bull et al., 2004).

Home visits to families with newborn babies are traditional services in many countries and provide the basis for future collaboration between the family and the nurse (Hjälmhult, 2009; Jansson et al., 2001). In Norway, all families with newborn babies must be offered a home visit by a public health nurse about two weeks postpartum. In the public health nurses' work, the home visit to the newborn is given high priority. This is often the first contact between the family and the public health nurses, if they have not met each other during the pregnancy (Norwegian Directorate of Health, 2004). The home visit after birth has a long tradition in Norway, and is a well-rehearsed routine. A key task at the home visit is to support the parents' mastery of the parenting role (Hjälmhult, 2009; Norwegian

Directorate of Health, 2004). Early contact is even more important at present, when newly fledged mothers are discharged from the hospital after a very short time.

At the home visit, the public health nurse has the opportunity to get to know the parents and any siblings in their own home (Hjälmhult, 2009; Jansson et al., 2001). The aim of the home visit is to evaluate the child's condition, get to know the family, create contact and trust, and evaluate what kind of help and support the family might need. The public health nurse listens to the family's questions and their need for guidance with the child. There might be questions concerning the birth, breastfeeding, infant care, or the family situation. Breastfeeding guidance and support are central concerns at any home visit to families with a newborn child (Norwegian Directorate of Health, 2004). In addition, the public health nurse receives important information about the parents' living conditions, and observes the interaction between the child and the family (Hjälmhult, 2009; Jansson et al., 1998, 2001; Norwegian Directorate of Health, 2004). The mothers are more satisfied when the first meeting with public health nurses is at a home visit than at a well-baby clinic (Hjälmhult, 2009). As all the services connected to the well-baby clinic and the home visits occur on a voluntary basis, it is important to establish a relationship of trust with the parents (Hjälmhult, 2009; Norwegian Directorate of Health, 2004). To ask the mother how *she* feels at the first postnatal visit may be essential. At this time when most of the focus is on the new baby, most mothers will welcome the concern about how they are doing.

In the study by Glavin et al. (2009, 2010b), as part of the municipality's screening procedure the public health nurses paid extra attention to mental health among postpartum mothers at the home visit and provided general information about mental health problems that may occur in the postpartum period. Each family also received an information brochure at the first home visit about 2 weeks after the birth. The public health nurses encouraged the fathers to be at home during the home visit. The parents were also invited to contact the well-baby clinic about the mother's possible mental health problems before the appointment at 6 weeks postpartum (Glavin et al., 2009, 2010b). The public health nurses felt that the screening procedure was helpful to the parents in several ways, and they regarded the home visits as particularly valuable (Glavin et al., 2010c). At the home visit, the public health nurses informed the parents about postnatal depression and the screening procedure, and had a dialogue about the mother's mental health. The public health nurses had undergone specific training related to postnatal depression and had more knowledge about this condition. This fact, in addition to the information given in pregnancy and postpartum, the brochure and the invitation to contact the well-baby clinic before the next appointment, may account for the significant difference that was detected between the two groups in the study (Glavin et al., 2009, 2010b). This support and information might have prevented postpartum depressive symptoms in women. Other studies support the findings. Thus, Morrell et al. (2009a) and Brugha et al. (2011) reported a decrease in the depression score among women who received support from the health visitors. Dennis and Creedy (2004) found that home visits after birth by public health nurses or midwives helped to prevent postnatal depression. In another study testing the preventive effect of information about postnatal depression, Taiwanese women were sent a booklet on postnatal depression at 6 weeks postpartum. Compared with those who did not receive this booklet, these women had significantly lower EPDS scores at 3 months postpartum (Heh & Fu, 2003).

These studies suggest that support and information may have a preventive effect on postnatal depression in women. The public health nurses in the study by Glavin et al. (2009c) reported that they thought the focus on mental health problems gave the home visit an altogether different significance. The mothers gave positive reports, and many of the multiparous mothers expressed the wish that they had received this information and tool after their first birth. In the public health nurses' opinion, providing information about mental health and handing out the brochure at the first home visit served as a kind of primary prevention. According to Dennis and Creedy (2004), psychosocial and psychological interventions may be effective treatment strategies, which may also be used in the early postpartum period to prevent postnatal depression. Stern (2006) states that home visits seem to have a positive effect on a wide variety of mental health and other problems, and the nonspecific positive factors may lie in the relationship between the health practitioners and the family, especially the mother. A newly fledged mother needs a secure base and the health practitioner may fill the need for a secure attachment figure (Stern, 2006). The information and support given by health practitioners during the home visit seem to have a preventive effect on postnatal depression in women.

### 3.5 Psychosocial and psychological interventions as prevention

The importance of psychosocial interventions in preventing minor depression is particularly important, since research suggests that minor depressive symptomatology often precedes a major depressive episode. In a review of 21 studies of preventative interventions for postnatal depression, Boath et al. (2005) found several studies suggesting positive short-term effects of psychological or supportive interventions. Many different psychological or supportive interventions exist. Examples include interpersonal psychotherapy, cognitive-behavioural therapy, psychological debriefing, supportive interactions, continuity of care, antenatal identification and notification, early postpartum follow-up, flexible postpartum care, educational strategies, and relaxation with guided imagery (Dennis & Creedy, 2004). In this review, including 15 trials, Dennis and Creedy (2004) found that women who received a psychosocial intervention were as likely to develop postnatal depression as those receiving standard care. However, one promising intervention was intensive postpartum support provided by public health nurses or midwives. Recent studies suggest that receiving care from health practitioners (health visitors, public health nurses) trained in identification and psychological intervention methods prevents cases of postnatal depression (Brugha et al., 2011; Glavin et al., 2010b).

In the study by Glavin et al. (2010b), the following elements constituted the main content of the intervention procedure postpartum: (1) increased focus on maternal mental health at a home visit about two weeks after delivery, (2) identification of women with postnatal depression at 6 weeks postpartum with the EPDS and a clinical assessment by the public health nurses, (3) one counselling session by a public health nurse after the mothers had completed the EPDS at 6 weeks postpartum, (4) supportive counselling sessions for the depressed mothers, (5) openness about mental health issues at every visit to the well-baby clinic, and (6) a system for referral for further treatment in the municipality.

All mothers had one counselling session with a public health nurse after completing the EPDS at 6 weeks, with a focus on the women's mental health. A clinical assessment by the public health nurse, charting the woman's current condition, how serious her problems were, her "history" of mental health problems, and her wishes, was important for further follow-up. The women whom the public health nurses regarded as needing treatment were then offered further supportive counselling sessions with the nurses between 6 weeks and 3 months postpartum. The counselling took place at the well-baby clinic, and each woman was followed up by the same public health nurse during the entire period. Each supportive counselling session lasted about 30 minutes. The number of counselling sessions was individualized according to each woman's need after assessment by the public health nurses and in agreement with the woman (Glavin et al., 2010b).

The public health nurses were trained to use active listening and empathetic communication (non-directive counselling) as a method. Establishing a positive relationship between the woman and the nurse was considered important. The nurse acted as an understanding listener, helping the woman by providing advice and alternative interpretations of past events only when asked (Rogers 1951, 1980). The method focused on the woman's experience, reflections, and ability to manage her own problems. Some main elements were emphasized in the counselling: 1) to listen and try to understand how things were from the woman's point of view, 2) to check their own understanding of the situation with the woman if unsure, 3) to treat the woman with the utmost respect and regard, 4) to be self-aware, self-accepting, and open with the woman. If the nurse made the judgment that a woman needed further help for her depression, she was referred to the municipality's mental health team, which included psychologists who could treat women with serious depression (Glavin 2010a, 2010b).

Findings from the study by Glavin et al. (2010b) suggest that home visits with increased focus on mothers' mental health, screening at 6 weeks postpartum and supportive counselling by trained public health nurses decrease the level of postnatal depression in the year following childbirth. Other studies support these findings (Brugda et al., 2011; Morrell et al., 2009a, 2009b). Thus, early identification and intervention might improve long-term prognoses for most women. A major part of prevention is being informed about the risk factors and the condition. The primary health care services can play a key role in identifying and treating postnatal depression. Women should be screened by their health practitioner to determine their risk for developing postnatal depression and the health practitioner should be aware of the importance of being sensitive and aware of changes in the mother's condition at all visits to the well-baby clinic.

### 3.6 The father's role

The father has an important role in the postpartum period and is often the nearest person to support the newly fledged mother. It may therefore be very important for the father to be informed about mental conditions that may occur in the postpartum period. In the study by Glavin et al. (2010c), public health nurses stated that it was valuable that the fathers were at home when the nurse visited the family. The information from the public health nurses increased the parents' understanding that it is common for women to experience postnatal depression in the postpartum period. This may influence the relationship between the parents. Misri et al. (2000) showed that partners' support reduced depressive symptoms among postpartum women. According to Misri et al. (2000), it is important to realize that the father is important for the child when the mother has postnatal depression. Further research is needed on this topic.

Studies have found the male partners of depressed women have higher than normal rates of depression. A father's depression might have implications for his ability to support his partner and for the relationship with the infant. Marital problems are a risk factor both for depression during the couple's transition to parenthood, and for adverse child outcomes (Buist et al., 2002).

## 4. Conclusion

Screening instruments such as the EPDS provide a tool to identify women who are depressed, but can also be used as a starting point for discussions about the mothers' psychological condition. The EPDS is easy to score and easy for the mothers to complete, and health professionals identify postnatal depression more frequently using the tool.

Information and support may have a preventive effect on postnatal depression in women. Flexible, individualized postnatal care that is provided by a professional and that incorporates postnatal depression screening tools appears to be promising to prevent postnatal depression in women. Increased focus on mother's mental health during the first year postpartum also seems to have preventive effects on postnatal depression and parenting stress in women.

In several countries, the circumstances for following up postpartum women are satisfactory, and in many countries mothers receive a home visit by a midwife, health visitor or public health nurse after birth. In these countries, almost all women who have given birth have frequent contact with well-baby clinics or health centres during the first year of the child's life. It is important to be aware of the new cases of women likely to be suffering from postnatal depression in the first year postpartum, as depression is strongly related to parenting stress. Trained health practitioners have the opportunity to identify and treat postnatal depression in women, which can improve the quality of the services provided. If additional training of health practitioners and information to the parents at the home visit can improve the quality of the services and provide support to the parents, this would seem to be a worthwhile investment. The prevention and treatment of postnatal depression could make a significant difference in women's lives and the lives of their children and families.

## 5. References


Abidin, R. (1995). *Parenting Stress Index: Professional Manual* (3rd ed), Psychological Assessment Resources Inc. Florida.

American Psychiatric Association. (1994). *Diagnostic and statistical manual of mental disorders,* (4th ed), American Psychiatric Association, Washington DC.

Beck, CT., & Gable, RK. (2001). Further validation of the Postpartum Depression Screening Scale. *Nursing Research,* 50, 155–164.

Beck, CT. (2006). Postpartum depression: it isn't just the blues. *The American Journal of Nursing,* 106, 40-50, quiz 50-1.

Beck, CT., Gable, RK. (2000). Postpartum Depression Screening Scale: Development and psychometric testing. *Nursing Research,* 49, 272-82.

Berle, JØ., Aarre, TF., Mykletun, A., Dahl, AA., & Holsten, F. (2003). Screening for postnatal depression. Validation of the Norwegian version of the Edinburgh Postnatal

Depression Scale, and assessment of risk factors for postnatal depression. *Journal of Affective Disorders,* 76, 151–156.

Boath, E., Bradley, E., & Henshaw, C. (2005). The prevention of postnatal depression: A narrative systematic review. *Journal of Psychosomatic Obstetrics & Gynecology,* 26, 185–192.

Brockington, I. (2004a). Postpartum psychiatric disorder. *The Lancet,* 363, 303–310.

Brockington, I. (2004b). Diagnosis and management of post-partum disorders: a review. *World Psychiatry,* 3, 89–95.

Brodén, MB., (2004). *Graviditetens muligheder,* Akademiske forlag, København (in Danish).

Brown, S., Small, R., Faber, B., Krastev, A., & Davis, P. (2002). Early postnatal discharge from hospital for healthy mothers and term infants. *The Cochrane Database of Systematic Reviews,* 3. No. CD002958. DOI: 10.1002/14651858. CD002958.

Brugha, TS., Morrell, CJ., Slade, P., & Walters, SJ. (2011). Universal prevention of depression in women postnatally: cluster randomized trial evidence in primary care. *Psychol Med,* Apr, 41(4), 739-48.

Buist, AE., Barnett, BE., Milgrom, J., Pope, S., Condon, JT., Ellwood, DA., Boyce, PM., Austin MP., & Hayes BA. (2002). To screen or not to screen – that is the question in perinatal depression, *Medical Journal of Australia,* 177, 101–105.

Bull, J., McCormack, G., Swann, C., & Mulvihill, C. (2004). *Ante- and post-natal home visiting: a review of reviews,* (1st ed), Health Development Agency, London.

Campbell, SB., Brownell, CA., Hungerford, A., Spieker, SJ., Mohan, R. & Blessing, JS. (2004). The course of maternal depressive symptoms and maternal sensitivity as predictors of attachment security at 36 months. *Development and Psychopathology,* 16, 231–252.

Chabrol, H., Teissedre, F., Saint-Jean, M., Teisseyre, N., Sistac ,C., Michaud, C., & Rogé B. (2002). Detection, prevention and treatment of post-partum depression: a controlled study of 859 patients. *Encephale,* 28, 65-70

Chick, N., & Meleis, AI. (1986). Transitions: A nursing concern. In *Nursing research methodology,* Chinn P.L., ed, pp. 237-257, Aspen Publication, Boulder CO.

Cooper, PJ., & Murray, L. (1998). Postnatal depression, clinical review. *British Medical Journal,* 316, 1884–1886.

Cox, JL., & Holden, J. (2003). *Perinatal mental health: A guide to the Edinburgh Postnatal Depression Scale (EPDS),* Gaskell, London.

Cox, JL. (2004). Postnatal mental disorder: towards ICD-11. *World Psychiatry,* 3, 96–97.

Cox, JL., Holden, J., & Sagovsky, R. (1987). Detection of postnatal depression. Development of the 10-item Edinburgh Postnatal Depression Scale. *British Journal of Psychiatry,* 150, 782–786.

Coyle B. & Adams C. (2002). The Edinburgh Postnatal Depression Scale: Guidelines for its use as a part of a maternal mood assessment. *Community Practitioner,* 75, 395–395.

Davies B.R., Howells S. & Jenkins M. (2003). Early detection and treatment of postnatal depression in primary care. *Journal of Advanced Nursing,* 44, 248–55.

Deave, T., Johnson, D., & Ingram, J. (2008). Transition to parenthood: the needs of parents in pregnancy and early parenthood. *BMC Pregnancy Childbirth,* 8:30, DOI: 10.1186/1471-2393-8-30.

Dennis, CL., & Chung-Lee, L. (2006). Postpartum depression help-seeking barriers and maternal treatment preferences: a qualitative systematic review. *Birth,* 33, 323–331.

Dennis, CL., & Creedy D. (2004). Psychosocial and psychological interventions for preventing postpartum depression. *Cochrane Database of Systematic Reviews,* 18, CD001134. DOI: 10.1002/14651858.CD001134.pub2.

Dennis, CL. (2003). The effect of peer support on post partum depression: a pilot randomized controlled trial. *Canadian Journal of Psychiatry,* 48, 115-124.

Dennis, CL. (2004). Treatment of Postpartum Depression, Part 2: A Critical Review of Nonbiological Interventions. *Journal of Clinical Psychiatry,* 65, 1252-1265.

Dennis, CL. (2009). Preventing and treating postnatal depression. Comprehensive screening programmes and better organization of care are key. *British Medical Journal,* 338, a2975, doi: 10.1136/bmj.a2975.

Dennis, CL., Hodnett. E., Kenton. L., Weston. J., Zupancic. J., Stewart. DE., & Kiss. A. (2009). Effect of peer support on prevention of postnatal depression among high risk women: multisite randomised controlled trial. *British Medical Journal,* 338, a3064.

Dennis, CL., Janssen, PA., & Singer, J. (2004). Identifying women at-risk for postpartum depression in the immediate postpartum period. *Acta Psychiatrica Scandinavica,* 110, 338-346.

Driscoll, JW. (2006). Postpartum depression: the state of the science. *Journal of Perinatal and Neonatal Nursing,* 20, 40–42.

Elliott, SA., Gerrard, J., Ashton, C., & Cox, JL. (2001). Training health visitors to reduce levels of depression after childbirth: An evaluation. *Journal of Mental Health,* 10, 613–625.

Evans, J., Heron, J., Francomb, H., Oke, S., & Golding, J. (2001). Cohort study of depressed mood during pregnancy and after childbirth. *British Medical Journal,* 323, 257-260.

Fitelson, E., Kim, S., Scott Baker, A., & Leight, K., (2011). Treatment of postpartum depression: clinical, psychological and pharmacological options. *International Journal of Women's Health,* 3 1–14, DOI: 10.2147/IJWH.S6938.

Freeman, MP., Wright, R., Watchman, M., Wahl, RA., Sisk, DJ., Fraleigh, L. & Weibrecht, JM. (2005). Postpartum depression assessments at well-baby visits: Screening feasibility, prevalence, and risk factors. *Journal of Women's Health,* 14, 929–935.

Gale, S., & Harlow, BL. (2003). Postpartum mood disorders: A review of clinical and epidemiological factors. *Journal of Psychosomatic and Obstetric Gynecology,* 24, 257-266.

Georgiopoulos, AM., Bryan, TL., Wollan, P., & Yawn, BP. (2001). Routine screening for Postpartum Depression. *Journal of Family Practice,* 50, 117–122.

Georgiopoulos, AM., Bryan, TL., Yawn, BP., Houston, MS., Rummans, TA., & Therneau, TM. (1999). Population-based screening for postpartum depression. *Obstetrics and Gynecology,* 93, 653–657.

Glavin, K., Ellefsen, B., & Erdal, B. (2010c). Norwegian Public Health Nurses' Experience in Using a Screening Protocol for Postpartum Depression. *Public Health Nursing,* 27, 255-261.

Glavin, K., Smith, L., & Sørum, R. (2009). Prevalence of postpartum depression in two municipalities in Norway. *Scandinavian Journal of Caring Sciences,* 23, 705-710.

Glavin, K., Smith, L., Sørum, R., & Ellefsen, B. (2010a). Supportive counseling by public health nurses for women with postpartum depression. *Journal of Advanced Nursing,* 66, 1317-1327.

Glavin, K., Smith, L., Sørum, R., & Ellefsen, B. (2010b). Redesigned community postpartum care to prevent and treat postpartum depression in women - a one year follow up study. *Journal of Clinical Nursing,* 19, 3051-62.

Gordon, TE., Cardone, IA., Kim, JJ., Gordon, SM., & Silver R.K. (2006). Universal perinatal depression screening in an Academic Medical Center. *Obstetrics & Gynecology,* 107, 342-347.

Halbreich, U., & Karkun, S. (2006). Cross-cultural and social diversity of prevalence of postpartum depression and depressive symptoms. *Journal of Affective Disorders,* 91, 97-111.

Heh, SS., & Fu, YY. (2003). Effectiveness of informational support in reducing the severity of postnatal depression in Taiwan. *Journal of Advanced Nursing,* 42, 30-36.

Hjälmhult, E. (2009). Skal helsesøster tilby hjemmebesøk til alle foreldre med nyfødt barn? *Sykepleien Forskning,* 4, 18–27 (in Norwegian).

Holland, WW., Stewart S., & Masseria C. (2006). *Policy brief: Screening in Europe,* World Health Organization 2006, On behalf of the European Observatory on Health Systems and Policies.

Horowitz JA., & Cousins, A. (2006). Postpartum depression treatment Rates for At-Risk Women. *Nursing Research,* 55, 23–27.

Horowitz, JA., & Goodman, JH. (2005). Identifying and Treating Postpartum Depression. *Journal of Obstetric, Gynecologic, and Neonatal Nursing,* 34, 264–273.

Jackson, C. (2007). The General Health Questionnaire. *Occupational Medicine,* 57, 79. doi:10.1093/occmed/kql169.

Jansson, A., Isacsson, A., Kornfält ,R., & Lindholm, LH. (1998). Quality in child healthcare. The views of mothers and public health nurses. *Scandinavian Journal of Caring Sciencies,* 12, 195-204.

Jansson, A., Petersson, K., & Uden, G. (2001). Nurses' first encounters with parents of new-born children--public health nurses' views of a good meeting. *Journal of Clinical Nursing,* 10, 140-151.

Kendall-Tacket, KA. (2005). *Depression in new mothers: Causes, consequences, and treatment alternatives,* Haworth Maltreatment and Trauma Press, New York.

Krantz, I., Eriksson, B., Lundquist-Persson, C., Ahlberg,BM., & Nilstun, T. (2008). Screening for postpartum depression with the Edinburgh Postnatal Depression Scale (EPDS): An ethical analysis. *Scandinavian Journal of Public Health,* 36, 211-216, DOI: 10.1177/1403494807085392.

Lanes, A., Kuk, JL., & Tamim, H. (2011). Prevalence and characteristics of Postpartum Depression symptomatology among Canadian women: a cross-sectional study. *BMC Public Health,* May 11.

Lee, DTS., Yip, ASK., Chiu, HFK., & Chung, KH. (2000). Screening for Postnatal Depression Using the Double-Test Strategy. *Psychosomatic Medicine,* 62, 258–263.

MacArthur, C., Winter, HR., Bick, DE., Lilford, R., Lancashire RJ., Knowles, H., Braunholtz, D.A., Henderson, C., Belfield, C., & Gee, H. (2003). Redesigning postnatal care: a randomised controlled trial of protocol-based midwifery-led care focused on individual women's physical and psychological health needs. *Health Technology Assessment,* 7, 1–98.

Mason, L., & Poole, H. (2008). Views of healthcare staff and mothers about postnatal depression screening. *Nursing Times,* 12, 44-47.

McLearn, KT., Minkovitz, CS., Strobino, DM., Marks, E., & Hou, W. (2006). Maternal depressive symptoms at 2 to 4 months postpartum and early parenting practices. *Archives of Pediatrics & Adolescent Medicine,* 16, 279–284.

Milgrom, J., Ericksen, J., Negri, L., & Gemmill, AW. (2005). Screening for postnatal depression in routine primary care: Properties of the Edinburgh Postnatal Depression Scale in an Australian sample. *Australian and New Zealand Journal of Psychiatry,* 39, 833–839.

Misri S., Kostaras X., Fox D., & Kostaras D. (2000). The impact of partner support in the treatment of postpartum depression. *The Canadian Journal of Psychiatry,* 45, 554–558.

Montazeri A., Torkan B., & Omidvari S. (2007). The Edinburgh Postnatal Depression Scale (EPDS): translation and validation study of the Iranian version. *BMC Psychiatry,* 4, 7-11.

Morrell, CJ., Slade, P., Warner, R., Paley, G., Dixon, S., Walters, SJ., Brugha, T., Barkham, M., Parry, GJ., & Nicholl, J. (2009b). Clinical effectiveness of health visitor training in psychologically informed approaches for depression in postnatal women: pragmatic cluster randomized trial in primary care. *British Medical Journal,* 338, a3045.

Morrell, CJ., Warner, R., Slade, P., Dixon, S., Walters, S., Paley, G., & Brugha, T. (2009a). Psychological interventions for postnatal depression: cluster randomised trial and economic evaluation. The PoNDER trial. *Health Technol Assess,* Jun;13(30):iii-iv, xi-xiii, 1-153.

Navarro, P., Ascaso, C., Garcia-Esteve, L., Aguado, J., Torres, A., & Martin-Santos, R. (2007). Postnatal psychiatric morbidity: a validation study of the GHQ-12 and the EPDS as screening tools. *General Hospital Psychiatry,* 29, 1-7.

Norwegian Directorate of Health. (2004). *The municipalities' work for health promotion and prevention in well baby clinics and school health services [Kommunenes helsefremmende og forebyggende arbeid i helsestasjons og skolehelsetjenesten],* Veileder til forskrift av 3. april 2003 nr. 450. Norway (in Norwegian).

O´Hara, MW. (1987). Post partum blues, depression and psychosis: a review. *Journal of Psykosomatic Obstretrics and Gynaecology,* 7, 205-227.

O'Hara, MV., & Swain, A.M. (1996). Rates and risk of postnatal depression—a meta-analysis. *International Review of Psychiatry,* 274, 740–743.

O'Hara, M.W., Zekoski, EM., Philipps, LH., & Wright EJ. (1990). Controlled prospective study of postpartum mood disorders: Comparison of childbearing and non-childbearing women. *Journal of Abnormal Psychology,* 99, 1–5.

O'Hara, MW., (1986). Social support, life events, and depression during pregnancy and the puerperium. *Archives of General Psychiatry,* 43, 569–573.

Olds, DL., Eckenrode, J., Charles, R., Henderson, J.; Kitzman, H., Powers, J., Cole, R., Sidora, K., Morris P., Pettitt, LM., & Luckey, D. (1997). Long-term Effects of Home Visitation on Maternal Life Course and Child Abuse and Neglect: Fifteen-year Follow-up of a Randomized Trial. *JAMA,* 278, 637-643.

Olds, DL., Robinson, J., O'Brien, R., Luckey, DW., Pettitt, LM., Henderson, CL., Rosanna, K., Sheff, KL., Korfmacher, J., Hiatt, S., & Talmi, A. (2002). Home Visiting by Paraprofessionals and by Nurses: A Randomized Controlled Trial. *Pediatrics,* 110, 486-496.

Poole, H., Mason, L., & Osborn, T. (2006). Women's views of being screened for postnatal depression. *Community Practitioner,* 79, 363–368.

Ray, KL., & Hodnett, ED. (2004). Caregiver support for postpartum depression (Cochrane Review). *The Cochrane Library,* Issue 1, 2004.

Rogers, CR. (1951). *Client-Centered Therapy,* Constable & Robinson, London.

Rogers, CR. (1980). *A Way of Being,* Houghton Mifflin Company, New York.

Rubertsson, C., Wickberg, B., Gustavsson, P., & Rådestad, I. (2005). Depressive symptoms in early pregnancy, two months and one year postpartum-prevalence and psychosocial risk factors in a national Swedish sample. *Archives of Women's Mental Health,* 8, 97-104.

Seeley, S., Murray, L., & Cooper, P. (1996). The outcome for mothers and babies of health visitor intervention. *Health Visitor,* 69, 135–138.

Seeley, S. (2001). Strengths and Limitations of the Edinburgh Postnatal Depression Scale, In: *Postnatal depression and maternal mental health: A public health priority. Conference proceedings,* Community Practitioners' and Health Visitors' Association, London.

Segre, LS., O'Hara, MW., Arndt, S., & Beck, CT. (2010). Screening and counseling for postpartum depression by nurses: the women's views. *MCN Am J Matern Child Nurs,* Sep-Oct, 35(5), 280-5.

Snoek, JE., & Engedal, K. (2000). *Psykiatri. Kunnskap, forståelse, utfordringer,* Akribe, Oslo (in Norwegian).

Stern, DN., & Bruschweiler-Stern, N. (2000). *En mor blir til,* Fagbokforlaget, Bergen (in Norwegian).

Stern, DN. (2006). Introduction to the special issue on early preventive intervention and home visiting. *Infant Mental Health Journal,* 27, 1-4.

Stewart, DE., Robertson, E., Dennis CL., & Grace, S. (2004). An evidence-based approach to post-partum depression. *World Psychiatry* 2004 3, 97–98.

Vik, K., Aass, IM., Willumsen, AB., & Hafting, M. (2009). "It's about focusing on the mother's mental health": screening for postnatal depression seen from the health visitors' perspective--a qualitative study. *Scandinavian Journal of Public Health,* 37, 239-245.

Vivilaki, VG., Dafermos, V., Kogevinas, M., Bitsios, P., & Lionis, C. (2009). The Edinburgh Postnatal Depression Scale: translation and validation for a Greek sample. *BMC Public Health,* 9, 329, DOI: 10.1186/1471-2458-9-329.

Wheatley, SL. (2005). *Coping with postnatal depression,* Sheldon Press, London.

Wickberg, B., & Hwang, CP. (2003). *Post partum depression – nedstämthet och depression i samband med barnefödande. [Post-partum depression – dejection and depression associated with childbirth],* Statens folkhälsoinstitut, 2003:59 (in Swedish).

Wilkins, C. (2006). A qualitative study exploring the support needs of first-time mothers on their journey towards intuitive parenting. *Midwifery,* 22, 169-18.

Zubaran, C., Schumacher, M., Roxo, MR., & Foresti, K. (2010). Screening tools for postpartum depression: validity and cultural dimensions. *African Journal of Psychiatry,* 13, 357 -365.

# 2

# Prelude to Parenthood: The Impact of Anxiety and Depression During Pregnancy

Carol Cornsweet Barber
*University of Waikato*
*New Zealand*

## 1. Introduction

This book, and a substantial body of literature that has developed over the last 40 years, attest to the importance of recognizing and treating depression in women and their partners in the early months and years of their parenthood. Articles and books in the popular literature (Osmond, Wilkie, & Moore, 2002; Shields, 2005), as well as internet resources and public and professional education initiatives (e.g., www.mededppd.org; www.postpartum.net; www.marcesociety.com) have contributed to broader awareness of the pervasiveness and impact of postnatal depression, and perhaps begun to decrease some of the stigma attached to the experience. It is still the case, however, that most lay people and many health and maternity professionals still focus primarily on the mental health needs of mothers (and sometimes fathers) *after* the baby is born (Highet, Gemmill, & Milgrom, 2011).

Over the last decade or two, however, there has been increasing awareness on the impact of emotional distress *during* pregnancy – growing recognition that the incidence of depression during pregnancy is at least as high as it is postnatally (Faisal-Cury & Menezes, 2007; Marcus, 2009), that the majority of cases of postnatal depression begin during pregnancy (Heron et al., 2004), that anxiety during pregnancy is a significant predictor of postnatal depression (Austin, Tully, & Parker, 2007), and that anxiety and stress during pregnancy can have significant long-term effects on the physical and mental health and development of the child.

This chapter will provide an overview of the literature on depression and anxiety during pregnancy, including prevalence of symptoms and syndromes, studies on the impact of depression, anxiety, and stress on birth outcomes and child development, the mechanisms by which these effects may operate, approaches to treatment of anxiety and depression during pregnancy, and the evidence available on the efficacy of these treatments. Implications for health and public policy, clinical treatment, and research will be discussed.

## 2. Prevalence of emotional disorders during pregnancy

Historically, it was thought that women were protected against psychiatric disorder during pregnancy (Cohen et al., 2006); however, epidemiological data collected over the last decade has not supported that view. The question of whether childbearing confers *extra* risk for emotional disorders in women has produced contradictory results across both antenatal and postnatal periods (Robertson, Grace, Wallington, & Stewart, 2004). Some authors have argued that there is an increase in rates of depression (Marcus, 2009), while others have found similar rates among pregnant and postnatal women and matched controls (Uguz, Gezginc, Kayhan, Sarı, & Büyüköz, 2010; van Bussel, Spitz, & Demyttenaere, 2006). The confluence of psychosocial and biological stressors during these times might explain an increased incidence of disorders such as depression and anxiety. Of course, the question of whether women are *more* at risk perinatally than at other times in their lives, while interesting for understanding the epidemiology and possibly the aetiology of perinatal emotional disorders, is less crucial than understanding the predictors, consequences, and most effective modes of treatment for women struggling with these problems during a time which may or may not be particularly vulnerable for women, but which a preponderance of evidence is showing is particularly vulnerable for the developing child, and for the developing parent-child relationship (Halligan, Murray, Martins, & Cooper, 2007; Murray & Cooper, 1997).

### 2.1 Antenatal depression

Since the recognition of the importance of antenatal as well as postnatal depression, a number of studies have looked at the prevalence of depression among pregnant women in the developed and developing world. Prevalence rates vary because of a variety of methodological factors. Many studies use the Edinburgh Postnatal Depression Scale (EPDS), a brief, self-report measure intended to screen for depressive symptoms (Cox, Holden, & Sagovksy, 1987), omitting the somatic items in other depression inventories which might produce a spurious over-identification of depression among women in the perinatal period.

Although the EPDS is described as a screen for depression, it contains items such as "I have been anxious or worried for no good reason", and factor analyses of the scale have revealed factors for depression and anxiety (Bowen, Bowen, Maslany, & Muhajarine, 2008; Swalm, Brooks, Doherty, Nathan, & Jacques, 2010). It may be more appropriate to consider the EPDS a measure of "distress," the mix of depression and anxiety that so often occurs together (Mauri et al., 2010). Nevertheless, the majority of the items on the scale focus on experiences such as sadness, tearfulness, self-blame, and anhedonia, and most studies use the EPDS as a screen for, or indication of, depressive symptoms in the perinatal period.

The EPDS has been used widely across a variety of cultures, and has been well validated for use antenatally (Jomeen & Martin, 2007). A cutoff score of 13 is often used for these studies to indicate a high probability of significant depression. Between one quarter and one third of women in relatively under-resourced populations tend to score above this cut-off. For example, 27% of a group of inner-city Canadian pregnant women (Bowen & Muhajarine, 2006) and 27.5% of Turkish pregnant women in a semi-urban region (Golbasi, Kelleci, Kisacik, & Cetin, 2010) scored at or above 13, and in a separate study, 33% of urban and semi-urban Turkish women scored at or above 13 (Senturk, Abas, Berksun, & Stewart, 2011). In a study of Jamaican women attending a university hospital clinic, 27% in the first trimester, 22% in the second, and 25% in the third trimester scored at or above 13 on the EPDS (Pottinger, Trotman-Edwards, & Younger, 2009).

Lower rates have been found in an educationally and economically advantaged sample of Vietnamese women; in this group, 8% of women scored at or above 12 (Fisher, Tran, & Tran, 2007). Texeireira's group (Teixeira, Figueiredo, Conde, Pacheco, & Costa, 2009) used a lower cut-off of 10 or higher, and so is difficult to compare with the above studies, but in this Portugese sample of women attending obstetric appointments, they found that 22%, 21%, and 18% (by trimester) scored above this threshold, consistent with other studies that suggest somewhat lower rates of depressive symptoms among women in developed countries. A large nationwide study in Australia recently found rates of 8.9% at or above 13 on the EPDS (Milgrom et al., 2008), though these rates do vary across subpopulations, and psychosocial factors appear to play a significant role, as will be discussed below.

Studies which use structured diagnostic interviews, rather than self-report questionnaires, tend to find lower rates of depression. Using a two-step process with the EPDS as a screen, followed by a structured clinical interview, a Nigerian study found that 8.3% of semiurban pregnant women were diagnosed with major or minor depressive disorder (Adewuya, Ola, Aloba, Dada, & Fasoto, 2007). Using a structured interview alone, Felice and colleagues found that 14.8% of women attending an antenatal clinic in Malta in the second trimester, and 10% of women in the third trimester met criteria for a depressive disorder (Felice, Saliba, Grech, Cox, & Caleja, 2007).

Although most of the research and clinical attention has been on unipolar depression among antenatal and postnatal women, there is evidence that women with bipolar disorders are at increased risk of postnatal psychosis, and women who have depressive symptoms should be screened for bipolar disorder and monitored for elevated mood. However, there is no consensus on the most effective screening method, with a variety of possible tools but no one well validated in antenatal women (Chessick & Dimidjian, 2010).

The line between depressive and anxiety disorders in perinatal as well as general populations is often blurred; when the EPDS has been factor-analyzed, although there are separate factors corresponding to depression and anxiety, several items have moderate loadings on both factors (Swalm, et al., 2010). Some services refer to antenatal or postnatal "distress" rather than attempt to differentiate depression from anxiety, and often women report a mix of anxious and depressed symptoms. In one large study using structured interviews to assess anxiety and depression among pregnant women, one-third of the sample was found to have comorbid anxiety and depressive diagnoses, more than either those with anxiety alone (8.5%) or depression alone (20%)(Field et al., 2010).

## 2.2 Antenatal anxiety

As is the case with depression, estimated rates of anxiety can vary widely depending on the method and criteria used to identify cases. Many studies use symptom inventories such as the State Trait Anxiety Inventory (STAI) (Spielberger, Gorsuch, Lushene, Vagg, & Jacobs, 1983); these should be considered a screen for possible anxiety disorder, or an indication of the level of anxiety symptoms, rather than a clinical diagnosis of any particular anxiety disorder, and the rates of occurrence found using self-report screens are typically significantly higher than those found when a structured clinical interview using formal diagnostic criteria is used. This is not, however, to minimize the importance of measurement of symptoms of anxiety along a continuum. In fact, many of the studies of the consequences of antenatal distress, to be discussed below, use self-report instruments, and find a significant relationship between high scores on distress and various outcome measures, regardless of whether any criterion for clinical diagnosis has been met. Those women who meet criteria for formal diagnosis might be considered the "tip of the iceberg", and one of the important questions for clinicians and policy makers is how to most effectively identify those women who are in distress and could benefit from support, rather than focusing primarily on diagnostic criteria.

Using the Portugese version of the STAI, with a cut-off of 45, Teixeira and colleagues (Teixeira, et al., 2009) measured anxiety symptoms among women in the first, second, and third trimesters, and found rates of significant anxiety of 15%, 12%, and 18%, respectively. They also screened for depression with the EPDS, using a cut-off of 10 or greater, and combined this with the STAI-S to describe a subset of women who scored highly on both anxiety and depression, with rates of 11%, 8%, and 11% across the three trimesters. Thus, about one in ten women in this sample were experiencing high levels of both anxiety and depressive symptoms.

In Bangladesh in a largely rural population, 29% of pregnant women scored above 45 on the trait subtest of the STAI in third trimester (Nasreen, Kabir, Forsell, & Edhborg, 2011). A Brazilian study used a lower cut-off of 41, and found that 59.5% of women were identified as having high state anxiety, and 45.3% high trait anxiety, in the last half of pregnancy (Faisal-Cury, Menezes, Araya, & Zugaib, 2009). A review summarizing a variety of studies of rates of significant anxiety in Africa came up with an overall mean prevalence of 14.8% for antenatal anxiety disorders (Sawyer, Ayers, & Smith, 2010).

Rates of anxiety disorders assessed by structured interview were relatively low in women in Malta, with 4.4% in the second trimester, but the authors reported that "several" women had anxiety symptoms that did not meet criteria for Generalized Anxiety Disorder because they had been present only since the beginning of the pregnancy, which was a duration of less than six months (Felice, et al., 2007). This low rate may also have been affected by the timing of the study; a Turkish study using structured interviews (Uguz, et al., 2010) found that 15.5% of women in the first trimester, 7.6% in the second, and 24.2% of women in the third trimester met criteria for an anxiety disorder.

Posttraumatic stress disorder is an anxiety disorder that might be expected to be of particular concern during pregnancy, given its association with high physiological arousal. In women, the index trauma often includes sexual abuse, so that the experience of maternity care and the anticipation of childbirth and caring for an infant may be extremely destabilizing (Sperlich & Seng, 2008). One study, using DSM-IV diagnostic criteria gathered in a structured interview, found that 3% of a sample of urban American pregnant women met full criteria for PTSD. Women who had PTSD also had increased rates of substance use, panic disorder, and depressive disorders (Rogal et al., 2007).

Obsessive-compulsive disorder and the spectrum of obsessive-compulsive symptoms, similar to depression, have been studied and discussed clinically more with respect to the postnatal period than during pregnancy. Many women with postnatal depression or anxiety struggle with intrusive thoughts and other obsessive-compulsive symptoms (Abramowitz et al., 2010), and, in fact, some degree of intrusive thoughts about accidents or harm coming to the baby are frequently present in new parents in general (Fairbrother & Woody, 2008).

These thoughts, however, are often kept private and not revealed to either professional or informal support people, for fear of losing custody of the baby or suffering the stigma that revealing such thoughts can elicit (Barber, 2009). The incidence of obsessive thoughts and/or obsessive-compulsive disorder during pregnancy has been examined in two very different contexts, with different methods and results. Uguz and colleagues (Uguz, et al., 2010) used a structured diagnostic interview to compare rates of anxiety and mood disorders in a group of Turkish pregnant women with a comparison sample of nonpregnant women of comparable age and socioeconomic status. They found similar rates of disorders in both groups, with a total of 19.4% of pregnant women meeting criteria for a DSM-IV mood or anxiety disorder. The single most common anxiety disorder was OCD, with 5.2% of pregnant women meeting full diagnostic criteria. An American study used self-report measures as well as structured interviews to assess level of OCD and depressive symptoms as well as diagnostic status in a group of women presenting to a university hospital obstetric clinic (Chaudron & Nirodi, 2010). In this longitudinal study, of those who participated in the structured interview during pregnancy, 29% met criteria for OCD. This high rate may have been affected by a combination of factors, including selective attrition, characteristics of the clinic's population, and a small sample size, but it is suggestive that a significant subgroup of pregnant women do suffer from OCD symptoms that impair their functioning, and seem likely to have an impact on their pregnancy and mothering.

Research across a wide variety of populations, then, has found that a significant proportion of women suffer during pregnancy from depression, anxiety, or a combination of the two. In an attempt both to understand the factors that contribute to this distress, and to identify groups of women who might be most in need of support and services, many studies have examined the individual and contextual factors that are associated with antenatal distress.

## 3. Risk factors for distress in pregnancy

In a recent review of the western literature on risk factors for depression in pregnancy, Lancaster and colleagues (Lancaster et al., 2010) found that the strongest predictors of depression during pregnancy were antenatal anxiety, history of depression, stressful negative life events, poor relationship quality and lack of social support from the partner, relying on public health insurance (largely the public Medicaid system in the US) and unintended pregnancy. Consistent, but less strong relationships were found between depression and domestic violence. Studies were inconsistent in their findings about the relationship between depression and socioeconomic status, cigarette, alcohol, and drug use, age and ethnicity. The authors note that these risk factors are generally consistent with the literature on risk factors for postnatal depression, with the exception that socioeconomic status has been more often found to be predictive of depression in the postnatal literature. They suggest that the studies they reviewed tended to be somewhat homogeneous with respect to SES, and this may have limited the findings (Lancaster, et al., 2010); in addition, it is important to note that this review was limited to studies performed in the US, Canada, Europe, Australia, and New Zealand, and so was relatively homogeneous with respect to culture and contextual economic factors.

Recent studies of correlates of antenatal depression from countries such as Turkey (Golbasi, et al., 2010), Bangladesh (Nasreen, et al., 2011) and Nigeria (Adewuya, et al., 2007) have been consistent with these findings; factors such as social support and relationship status are consistently noted. Some studies (Adewuya, et al., 2007; Golbasi, et al., 2010) have found history of stillbirth to be associated with depression, but this was not consistently found in the Lancaster review, possibly because of the relative rarity of this event, particularly in well-resourced countries.

The literature on risk for anxiety during pregnancy is less well-developed, but studies of prevalence of antenatal anxiety and/or distress often note many of the same risk factors as have been found for antenatal depression. For example, one study in Turkey looked at factors associated with a measure of mixed anxiety and depression, and found that poverty and partner unemployment, domestic violence, and unwanted pregnancy predicted distress (Karmaliani et al., 2009). Intimate partner violence, as well as sexual coercion, were associated with symptoms of PTSD as well as depression in an Indian study (Varma, Chandra, Thomas, & Carey, 2007). A longitudinal study of distress and relationship adjustment during pregnancy found that relationship adjustment was correlated with concurrent anxiety and depression, and that poor relationship adjustment predicted subsequent anxiety during and after pregnancy (Whisman, Davila, & Goodman, 2011).

Using data from the Avon Longitudinal Study of Parents and Children (ALSPAC), researchers were able to look at the association between self-reported history of eating disorders and other psychiatric disorders on the risk of experiencing significant anxiety and depression during pregnancy, and found that history of depression or past or current eating disorder conferred an increased risk of anxiety and depression perinatally (Micali, Simonoff, & Treasure, 2011). Looking more specifically at generalized anxiety disorder, Buist, Gotman and Yonkers (2011) found that history of GAD, less education, lower social support, and history of child abuse were associated with GAD symptoms during pregnancy.

Across types of antenatal distress, then, history of emotional disorders is the strongest and most consistent predictor of distress, and so women who have a history of depression or anxiety and become pregnant are clearly a group who should be monitored and provided support. In addition, various aspects of social and interpersonal relationships are associated with risk, and women with abusive, distant, or conflicted relationships are more likely to suffer distress. Conversely, women in supportive, stable relationships, or who have a network of family and friends they can rely on, are less likely to struggle during this time. Fewer studies have looked for protective factors or individual strengths that might help women to cope with the stresses of pregnancy, but there is some evidence that characteristics such as secure attachment (van Bussel, Spitz, & Demyttenaere, 2009), confidence (Edwards, Galletly, Semmler-Booth, & Dekker, 2008) and optimism (Grote, Bledsoe, Larkin, Lemay, & Brown, 2007) are associated with lower levels of distress.

## 4. Consequences of stress and distress in pregnancy

Antenatal stress and distress are common, and are especially prevalent among certain vulnerable populations, so that it may be possible to identify and focus efforts at intervention. The case for investing resources in women and families early in the parenting experience is strong because what is at stake is not only the mental health and well-being of the women involved, but also the impact that antenatal distress can have on the developing fetus and the developing caregiving relationship. Evidence has been accumulating from both animal and human studies that there are serious and long lasting effects of psychological distress during pregnancy.

Animal research has been largely on the impact of stress on development, and a wide variety of studies have found that antenatal stress, particularly stress in which the animal has little control over the stressor (e.g., restraint, loud noise), produces a significant increase in stress hormones, which, in turn, have an effect on brain development, cardiovascular health, and behavioural problems in offspring (Charil, Laplante, Vaillancourt, & King, 2010; Harris & Seckl, 2011).

Research on antenatal stress and distress in humans has found that both depression and stress are consistently associated with increased rates of adverse birth outcomes such as preterm delivery, low birthweight, and fetal growth retardation (Diego et al., 2009; Field, Diego, & Hernandez-Reif, 2006; Littleton, Bye, Buck, & Amacker, 2010; Uguz, Gezginc, & Yazici, 2011). In addition, infants born to mothers with depression have been found to have higher levels of cortisol and lower levels of dopamine and serotonin than comparison infants, and also showed more restless sleep, more relative right frontal EEG (an indicator of negative mood), and less optimal neurobehavioral indicators on the Brazelton Neonatal Behavior Assessment Scale (Field et al., 2004). In general, infants born to depressed or distressed mothers are vulnerable on a variety of developmental and social measures, suggesting that they may be more difficult to sooth and care for than other infants (Field, Diego, et al., 2006). This challenge compounds the already difficult task of the new mother who is likely to be continuing her struggle with emotional distress.

## 5. Mechanisms for understanding impact of antenatal stress and distress

Results of animal and human research have suggested a variety of mechanisms by which antenatal stress and distress may have an impact on infant health and development. Physiologically, maternal stress and mood changes are associated with hormonal and neurotransmitter changes, and parallel changes can be observed in the offspring of pregnant women with depression (Charil, et al., 2010; Field, et al., 2004). The stress hormone cortisol, which increases under a variety of stressful circumstances, is also intimately involved with the developmental processes of the fetus, for example, being necessary to the process of preparing the fetal lungs for functioning (Charil, et al., 2010). Chronic high levels of maternal cortisol are transmitted to the infant, and may affect infant brain development in areas including the hippocampus, amygdala, hypothalamus, neocortex, cerebellum, and corpus callosum (Charil, et al., 2010). Stress also affects the functioning of the placenta, which may be the mechanism of some of the effects of maternal stress on neurodevelopment (Charil, et al., 2010).

In addition to this direct effect of maternal stress on fetal development, antenatal depression and anxiety may affect the woman's self-care and health behaviors, which in turn have an impact on the child. Emotional distress, and depression in particular, may make it more difficult for women to access antenatal health care, to monitor their diet to ensure appropriate nutrition, and to refrain from smoking, alcohol use, and the use of other drugs that may serve a self-soothing function. One study that looked at various aspects of stress in pregnancy found that high levels of stress and anxiety were associated with smoking, caffeine use, and unhealthy eating, and that there was a direct association between pregnancy-specific stress (i.e., worry about specific aspects of the pregnancy) and pre-term delivery, and also an indirect association between pregnancy-specific stress and low birth weight, mediated by cigarette smoking (Lobel et al., 2008).

Antenatal distress is also the strongest, most consistent predictor of postnatal depression across a variety of populations and study methods (Grant, McMahon, & Austin, 2009; Heron, O'Connor, Evans, Golding, & Glover, 2004; Kirpinar, Gozum, & Pasinlioglu, 2010; Milgrom, et al., 2008; Robertson, et al., 2004). Postnatal depression has been shown in longitudinal studies to be associated with significant cognitive, emotional, and behavioural difficulties in children (Halligan, et al., 2007; Murray & Cooper, 1997). Some of the effect of maternal distress is likely mediated by caregiving behaviors such as sensitivity and availability (Grant, McMahon, Reilly, & Austin, 2010), and the effect that depression and anxiety may have on the mother's confidence in parenting and developing attachment with the infant (Dayton, Levendosky, Davidson, & Bogat, 2010).

## 6. Interventions to support women and families

Although there has been a good deal of work done to develop and test interventions to prevent and treat postnatal depression (Kopelman & Stuart, 2005), there is less systematic investigation of the effectiveness of interventions for antenatal depression, and even less work with respect to anxiety. However, there are a number of promising approaches that have been developed and applied to women during the antenatal period. These approaches vary considerably, including medical, psychological, lifestyle, spiritual, and psychoeducational strategies, with varying levels of intensity and commitment of resources. This variety is potentially a strength for the field, providing an array of options for helping women and families so that the woman, perhaps in consultation with a health, mental health, or maternity care provider, can choose a set of tools to try that is tailored to her particular level of distress, practical situation, and expectations and beliefs about what is most likely to help.

The great variety of traditional and complementary approaches to addressing distress in pregnancy probably stems in part from the multidisciplinary nature of perinatal care, which involves physicians, midwives, nurses, social workers, psychologists, and others, each providing different theoretical models of understanding health and mental health. In addition, childbearing is a normative experience that joins people from all cultures and traditions, and helping women who struggle at this time is a longstanding need and concern, even when it is not recognized in formal mental health terms. The contributions of all of these perspectives make for a rich mix of potential approaches, but it can also be a challenge to sort the wheat from the chaff, to identify which strategies are most likely to be helpful, and what the risks might be, either from negative side effects of an active treatment, or from choosing a treatment that is ineffective and in doing so, losing an opportunity during a critical time.

In considering options for treatment during pregnancy, it is important first to consider the level of distress the woman is experiencing, and risk (and opportunity) this entails. Where there is severe distress, and the intensity of the painful feelings are such that the woman feels driven to escape through suicide or substance use, a commensurate response with intensive treatment, possibly hospitalization, probably medication, and engagement with the partner and other support network is likely to be necessary (Choate & Gintner, 2011; Yonkers et al., 2009). However, in most cases, this intensity of treatment is not necessary or practical. Many women who have moderate to severe distress according to their responses on screening questionnaires do not consider themselves to be "depressed," and will not accept a referral to an unfamiliar mental health service (Carter et al., 2005; Miller, Shade, & Vasireddy, 2009). On the other hand, woman often do not consider their maternity care provider to be the appropriate person to talk to about their psychological distress (Bennett et al., 2009), and in the end, the majority of women with significant depression during pregnancy receive no mental health services at all (Flynn, Blow, & Marcus, 2006; Smith et al., 2009). This is not to say that they do not receive any support for their distress; they may seek support from friends, family, clergy, midwives, childbirth educators, and others (Barber, 2008). The number and popularity of books and websites on pregnancy and childbearing testify to the number who use informational support to cope with stress and uncertainty.

The array of options for support for women with antenatal distress includes self-help resources such as books and websites, support groups, clergy and religious community, visiting nurses, midwives, and health workers, complementary medicine providers, mental health providers, and medical professionals. It has been suggested that one of the barriers to universal screening for perinatal depression in obstetric or midwifery practice is the possibility of uncovering cases of serious distress, without the back-up of prompt accessible mental health services (Miller, et al., 2009). It is unrealistic, both in terms of cost and workforce, to expect to be able to provide formal mental health services to the 20-30% of the pregnant population who might score above a screening threshold for anxiety or depression. However, if front-line maternity providers have awareness and basic knowledge of the importance of attending to stress and distress in pregnancy, and have available to them an array of options and some tools with which to help women choose among the approaches, then it is possible that more of this distress will be recognized and ameliorated, and those who need mental health services may be more likely to get them.

The following sections will provide an overview of the array of options for prevention and intervention that have been examined empirically, and for which there seems to be some support. This list is not exhaustive; there may be many traditional or innovative interventions that are potentially useful, but have not been subjected to research or discussed in the psychological literature.

### 6.1 Preventative interventions and strategies

A few studies have described interventions that have potential to help women manage stress and anxiety, entail virtually no risk, and are targeted at all pregnant women or, in the case of physical exercise, may exclude some women with physical complications that restrict their activity levels. Lox and Treasure (Lox & Treasure, 2000), for example, examined the effect of aqua exercise on pregnant women who participated twice a week for six weeks; they found an increase in well-being, and decreases in distress and fatigue following the exercise. This was a self-selected group who chose to participate in the exercise programme, but there is considerable evidence that exercise can improve mood and anxiety (Shivakumar et al., 2011), and that levels of physical activity tend to decrease during pregnancy (Poudevigne & O'Connor, 2006). There have been no systematic studies of the effects of exercise on depression during pregnancy, but this is a promising area (Shivakumar, et al.,

2011). The challenge, as ever, is how to help women, especially depressed women, to participate consistently in an exercise programme. It may be helpful to consider adding a social component to an exercise programme, such as walking with a group or a friend (Armstrong & Edwards, 2004).

Specific forms of exercise, combined with meditation and/or spiritual components, have also been used with pregnant women. Yoga classes specifically for pregnant women are popular in many areas, and yoga has been found to have a positive effect on birth outcomes (Beddoe & Lee, 2008) as well as ratings of stress and anxiety (Beddoe, Paul Yang, Kennedy, Weiss, & Lee, 2009). Qi exercise is similar to yoga, and involves stretching, breathing, and meditation; one study compared a group of women who participate in 12 weeks of twice-weekly Qi sessions with a control group, and found that the Qi group had lower physical discomfort and depressive symptoms, but there was no significant difference in anxiety between the groups (Ji & Han, 2010).

Music therapy has been proposed as a low-cost, low-risk intervention for managing stress and distress, and one study found a significant decrease, compared with a randomized control group, on stress, anxiety, and depression, after two weeks of 30 minutes per day of listing to selected music (Chang, Chen, & Huang, 2008).

There have also been a number of studies that have provided interventions to women with high antenatal distress, in an attempt to prevent postnatal depression. Most of these studies have found few or no significant treatment effects (Austin et al., 2008; Lara, Navarro, & Navarrete, 2010; Milgrom, Schembri, Ericksen, Ross, & Gemmill, 2011); however, Milgrom's group has developed an intervention that involves a combination of a self-help book for women and weekly telephone support to structure and complement the bibiotherapy. This intervention did produce a significant reduction of depression, anxiety, and stress, and a decreased percentage of women who were above threshold for depression postnatally (Milgrom, et al., 2011).

### 6.2 Psychological and biological treatments

Formal psychotherapy has been well studied for postnatal depression, and both Cognitive Behavior Therapy (CBT) and Interpersonal Therapy (IPT) have been found to be effective, but the results of the few studies of antenatal psychotherapy have been less clear (Choate & Gintner, 2011). Studies of CBT delivered antenatally have been equivocal (Choate & Gintner, 2011), although one recent study found some positive effect of a group CBT during pregnancy (Le, Perry, & Stuart, 2011). Interpersonal therapy has been more consistently successful in pregnancy; a randomized controlled trial showed significant improvements in mood for pregnant women provided with IPT (Spinelli & Endicott, 2003), and Grote has adapted IPT to be briefer and specifically tailored to the needs of economically stressed minority women (Grote et al., 2009), and found positive effects on depression during and after pregnancy, and on postnatal social functioning.

Although most women, when asked their preferences for treatment for depression during pregnancy, prefer psychotherapy over medication (Kim et al., 2011), there are times when medication may be required for effective treatment (Yonkers, et al., 2009). There are no randomized controlled trials of medication treatment of antenatal depression (Gentile & Galbally, 2011), but many women are treated with medications during pregnancy, and professional guidelines suggest that the woman and her doctor need to carefully weigh the (unknown) risks of medication against the (known and unknown) risks of depression during pregnancy (Yonkers, et al., 2009). A recent review of the effects of antidepressant medication during pregnancy on neurodevelopment in the child concluded that there are too many methodological problems in the existing studies to draw firm conclusions, but there are no studies showing clear longstanding negative effects of medication (Gentile & Galbally, 2011).

It has been suggested that transcranial magnetic stimulation (TMS) might be an effective option for women with moderate to severe depression who prefer not to take medication during pregnancy (Kim, et al., 2011); however, there has been no research on the safety or efficacy of this treatment during pregnancy, and when pregnant women were asked whether they would consider this treatment, which involves daily office visits for four weeks, only 16% said they would consider it as an option if they needed mental health treatment (Kim, et al., 2011).

Supplements such as SAMe and St. John's Wort have been used postnatally and there is some evidence of efficacy, but not enough information on safety antenatally to recommend treatment (Freeman, 2009). Omega-3 fatty acids do seem to be safe and generally beneficial to health and development in pregnancy, and results on treatment for depression are somewhat mixed but promising, especially in conjunction with other therapies (Freeman, 2009; Freeman et al., 2008).

Bright light therapy has had positive effects with depression outside of pregnancy, and a few small studies have suggested it is promising for antenatal depression with relatively low risk (Freeman, 2009), though one study did report a case of hypomania triggered by bright light, pointing up the need for awareness and assessment of bipolar disorder (Chessick & Dimidjian, 2010).

Acupuncture is a traditional treatment that has been used for depression; most of the research literature is difficult to evaluate from a western perspective because it is published in Asian languages and represents different models of diagnosis and research (Freeman, 2009). However, one small randomized controlled trial compared acupuncture with massage, and found decreased rates of depression in the group treated with a depression-specific acupuncture protocol (Manber, Schnyer, Allen, Rush, & Blasey, 2004).

Several studies have suggested that massage during pregnancy, particularly moderate pressure massage, reduces depression and anxiety and lowers cortisol levels (Field, Diego, & Hernandez-Reif, 2010; Field, Diego, Hernandez-Reif, Deeds, & Figueiredo, 2009). When massage is provided by the woman's partner, not only does her mood improve, but the partner's as well, and there is an increase in ratings of relationship quality (Field, Diego, & Hernandez-Reif, 2010). This research group has also reported that infants of depressed mothers who receive massage during pregnancy have more favorable neurobehavioral profiles than a comparison group (Field, Hernandez-Reif, & Diego, 2006).

It seems possible that at least part of the effect of interventions such as massage, meditation, and music therapy are mediated by a state of relaxation; a few studies have found an immediate positive impact of relaxation on mood (Urech et al., 2010) and fetal response (Fink et al., 2011); however, this may be more complex in clinical samples. One study found less effect of a single session of relaxation in women who were highly anxious than in those with lower anxiety (Alder, Urech, Fink, Bitzer, & Hoesli, 2011). There are no controlled studies of clinical relaxation training in distressed pregnant women, but this seems a promising area for investigation.

Biofeedback can be used as a tool for teaching relaxation, and has been shown to have a positive effect in decreasing frequency of migraines during pregnancy (Airola et al., 2010). Biofeedback teaches control over physiological processes that initially seem out of conscious control. There is some evidence that the magnitude of the physiological stress response is related to the extent to which the individual has control over the stressor (Charil, et al., 2010), and in a stressful situation, women who see themselves as having more control over the stress are less vulnerable to depression (Grote, et al., 2007). For this reason, biofeedback, perhaps combined with some cognitive interventions to help women to assess their situation and identify the most effective coping strategies, might be a particularly effective intervention during pregnancy, when many women experience their body and the process of medical care during pregnancy as being out of control.

## 7. Conclusion

The antenatal period presents an opportunity, when women and their partners are at a point of disequilibrium, reorganizing their perspectives, priorities, and relationships in order to make way for the new family member. This can represent a crisis, but also may be a point at which they are open to change, and are in contact with systems and services that might be supportive to positive change. Interventions that use natural relationships and supports and build those relationships, such as training partners to provide massage (Field, et al., 2009), seem particularly promising, perhaps along with encouraging women to choose among various methods of relaxation (e.g., music, biofeedback, meditation, guided imagery), and exercise (aqua exercise, walking, yoga, Qi, etc). These are low cost, low risk ideas that could be promoted for all pregnant women, and perhaps offered with more support and prompting to women who show signs of mild to moderate distress.

For women who are clearly struggling with significant levels of depression and/or anxiety, encouraging social support and self-care, as above, may need to be augmented with brief psychotherapy such as ITP-B (Grote, et al., 2009). This model may be particularly appropriate because the emphasis on assessing and addressing relationship problems has the best chance of helping women who are in abusive or conflicted relationships, given the consistent links between perinatal distress and social support, relationship quality, and domestic violence.

If the level or nature of the anxiety and/or depression is such that the woman does not get relief from psychosocial strategies, and the distress is impacting her functioning and self-care, there is significant risk to the baby and to the mother's long-term wellbeing, and she may be encouraged to consider medication. Ideally, she will have an ongoing relationship with a therapist who can help the woman and her partner to consider treatment options and make choices that fit with their values and expectations, and to feel empowered, rather than overwhelmed and disempowered, by the experience of choice. In this instance, it seems wise to invest resources in an ongoing relationship with a therapist who knows the family well and can help the vulnerable mother to manage the transition to parenthood, recognizing and supporting her strengths and providing emotional support, perspective, information, and problem-solving skills. Postnatally, then, the therapist can be alert to needs and issues as they arise, both in the mother's mood and functioning, and also assessing and fostering sensitivity and attunement to the infant's needs (Grant, et al., 2010).

There is considerable promise in the richness of support and diversity of approaches that can be offered to women during pregnancy, but there are also significant barriers that must be acknowledged and addressed in order to promote the wellbeing of developing families. For many people, the stigma of being labelled "depressed" or of accessing mental health services is daunting, and they are unwilling to make use of help that requires them to adopt the role of patient in a mental health setting. This may be part of the reason such a small proportion of women with significant depression access services, and in planning services, it is important to consider the language used and the location of the services in order to make them more accessible and acceptable to the women who need them. It is also important to acknowledge the realities of the lives of women who are struggling during pregnancy; many are poor, have other children, and have limited transportation and time; services that tailor their approach to the realistic needs of their clients, and which are respectful of the culture and context of the women they serve, are more likely to be successful (Grote, et al., 2009). This applies as much to the array of complementary and preventative services as to psychotherapy. Recommending yoga to a poor single parent with three children under five is unlikely to be successful, but taking the time to get to know the woman, and finding out whether she might be able to listen to music, attend church services, or arrange to walk with a friend, may be to take a step with her toward more effective self-care, in hopes that this will enable her to be more emotionally balanced and available to her children.

This chapter has focused almost exclusively on the problems and needs of pregnant women; it is important to recognize and address, as well, the problems and needs of the partners of pregnant women, who are also grappling with many changes during the transition to parenthood (Boyce, Condon, Barton, & Corkindale, 2007; Genesoni & Tallandini, 2009). Development of intervention strategies that include partners, and acknowledge their needs, is an area of growing interest , but one in which there is relatively little research so far.

Pregnancy is a time of transition, and is ripe with risk, but also with opportunity. It is a time when those who serve women and families must be alert to distress, and sensitive to the social pressures that may lead women to hide their distress and to dismiss their own needs. A woman's needs at this time are inseparable from her baby's needs, and the needs of society are served by providing support and care to all developing families.

## 8. Acknowledgements

The author wishes to acknowledge my colleagues Nicola Starkey, Beverly Burns, Neville Robertson, and Kyle Smith for their contributions and support.

## 9. References

Abramowitz, j. S., Meltzer-Brody, S., Leserman, J., Killenberg, S., Rinaldi, K., Mahaffey, B. L., & Pederson, C. (2010). Obsessional thoughts and compulsive behaviors in a sample of women with postpartum mood symptoms. *Archives of Women's Mental Health, 13,* 523-530.

Adewuya, A. O., Ola, B. A., Aloba, O. O., Dada, A. O., & Fasoto, O. O. (2007). Prevalence and correlates of depression in late pregnancy among Nigerian women. *Depression and anxiety, 24,* 15-21.

Airola, G., Allais, G., Castagnoli Gabellari, I., Rolando, S., Mana, O., & Benedetto, C. (2010). Non-pharmacological management of migraine during pregnancy. *Neurol Sci, 31 Suppl 1,* S63-65. 1590-3478 (Electronic) 1590-1874 (Linking).

Alder, J., Urech, C., Fink, N., Bitzer, J., & Hoesli, I. (2011). Response to induced relaxation during pregnancy: comparison of women with high versus low levels of anxiety. *J Clin Psychol Med Settings, 18*(1), 13-21. 1573-3572 (Electronic) 1068-9583 (Linking).

Armstrong, K., & Edwards, H. (2004). The effectiveness of a pram-walking exercise programme in reducing depressive symptomatology for postnatal women. *Int J Nurs Pract, 10*(4), 177-194. 1322-7114 (Print) 1322-7114 (Linking).

Austin, M.-P., Frilingos, M., Lumley, J., Hadzi-Pavlovic, D., Roncolato, W., Acland, S., . . . Parker, G. (2008). Brief antenatal cognitive behaviour therapy group intervention for the-prevention of postnatal depression and anxiety: A randomised controlled trial. *Journal of Affective Disorders, 105*(1-3), 35-44. 0165-0327.

Austin, M.-P., Tully, L., & Parker, G. (2007). Examining the relationship between antenatal anxiety and postnatal depression. *Journal of Affective Disorders, 101,* 169-174.

Barber, C. C. (2008). *Supports and services for early parenting in Hamilton, New Zealand: an exploration of the experiences of mothers and fathers.* Paper presented at the Biannual meeting of the Marce Society: Policy, Planning and Effective Delivery of Perinatal Mental Health Care, Sydney, Australia.

Barber, C. C. (2009). Perinatal mental health care in New Zealand: the promise of beginnings. *New Zealand Journal of Psychology, 38*(1), 32-38.

Beddoe, A. E., & Lee, K. A. (2008). Mind-body interventions during pregnancy. *J Obstet Gynecol Neonatal Nurs, 37*(2), 165-175. 0884-2175 (Print) 0090-0311 (Linking).

Beddoe, A. E., Paul Yang, C. P., Kennedy, H. P., Weiss, S. J., & Lee, K. A. (2009). The effects of mindfulness-based yoga during pregnancy on maternal psychological and physical distress. *J Obstet Gynecol Neonatal Nurs, 38*(3), 310-319. 1552-6909 (Electronic) 0090-0311 (Linking).

Bennett, I. M., Palmer, S., Marcus, S., Nicholson, J. M., Hantsoo, L., Bellamy, S., . . . Coyne, J. C. (2009). "One end has nothing to do with the other:" patient attitudes regarding help seeking intention for depression in gynecologic and obstetric settings. *Arch Womens Ment Health, 12*(5), 301-308. 1435-1102 (Electronic).

Bowen, A., Bowen, R., Maslany, G., & Muhajarine, N. (2008). Anxiety in a socially high-risk sample of pregnant women in Canada. *The Canadian Journal of Psychiatry, 53*(7), 435-440.

Bowen, A., & Muhajarine, N. (2006). Prevalence of antenatal depression in women enrolled in an outreach program in Canada. *Journal of Obstetric, Gynecological and Neonatal Nursing, 35,* 491-498.

Boyce, P., Condon, J., Barton, J., & Corkindale, C. (2007). First-Time Fathers' Study: psychological distress in expectant fathers during pregnancy. *Aust N Z J Psychiatry, 41*(9), 718-725. 0004-8674 (Print) 0004-8674 (Linking).

Carter, F. A., Carter, J. D., Luty, S. E., Wilson, D. A., Frampton, C. M. A., & Joyce, P. R. (2005). Screening and treatment for depression during pregnancy: a cautionary note. *Australian and New Zealand Journal of Psychiatry, 39*(4), 255-261. 0004-8674.

Chang, M. Y., Chen, C. H., & Huang, K. F. (2008). Effects of music therapy on psychological health of women during pregnancy. *J Clin Nurs, 17*(19), 2580-2587. 1365-2702 (Electronic) 0962-1067 (Linking).

Charil, A., Laplante, D. P., Vaillancourt, C., & King, S. (2010). Prenatal stress and brain development. *Brain Res Rev, 65*(1), 56-79. 1872-6321 (Electronic) 0165-0173 (Linking).

Chaudron, L. H., & Nirodi, N. (2010). The obsessive-compulsive spectrum in the perinatal period: a prospective pilot study. *Archives of Women's Mental Health, 13*, 403-410.

Chessick, C. A., & Dimidjian, S. (2010). Screening for bipolar disorder during pregnancy and the postpartum period. *Arch Womens Ment Health, 13*(3), 233-248. 1435-1102 (Electronic).

Choate, L. H., & Gintner, G. G. (2011). Prenatal Depression: Best Practice Guidelines for Diagnosis and Treatment. *Journal of Counseling and Development, 89*(3), 373-381. 0748-9633.

Cohen, L. S., Altshuler, L. L., Harlow, B. L., Nonacs, R., Newport, D. J., Viguera, A. C., . . . Stowe, Z. N. (2006). Relapse of major depression during pregnancy in women who maintain or discontinue antidepressant treatment. *JAMA, 295*(5), 499-507. 1538-3598 (Electronic) 0098-7484 (Linking).

Cox, J., Holden, J., & Sagovksy, R. (1987). Detection of postnatal depression: development of the 10-item Edinburgh Postnatal Depression Scale. *British Journal of Psychiatry, 150*, 782-786.

Dayton, C. J., Levendosky, A. A., Davidson, W. S., & Bogat, G. A. (2010). The child as held in the mind of the mother: the influence of prenatal maternal representations on parenting behaviors. *Infant Mental Health Journal, 31*(2), 220-241.

Diego, M. A., Field, T., Hernandez-Reif, M., Schanberg, S., Kuhn, C., & Gonzalez-Quintero, V. H. (2009). Prenatal depression restricts fetal growth. *Early Hum Dev, 85*(1), 65-70. 1872-6232 (Electronic) 0378-3782 (Linking).

Edwards, B., Galletly, C., Semmler-Booth, T., & Dekker, G. (2008). Antenatal psychosocial risk factors and depression among women living in socioeconomically disadvantaged suburbs in Adelaide, South Australia. *Australian and New Zealand Journal of Psychiatry, 42*, 45-50.

Fairbrother, N., & Woody, S. (2008). New mothers' thoughts of harm related to the newborn. *Archives of Women's Mental Health, 11*, 221-229.

Faisal-Cury, A., Menezes, P., Araya, R., & Zugaib, M. (2009). Common mental disorders during pregnancy: prevalence and associated factors among low-income women in Sao Paulo, Brazil: depression and anxiety during pregnancy. *Arch Womens Ment Health, 12*(5), 335-343. 1435-1102 (Electronic).

Faisal-Cury, A., & Menezes, P. R. (2007). Prevalence of anxiety and depression during pregnancy in a private setting sample. *Archives of Women's Mental Health, 10*, 25-32.

Felice, E., Saliba, J., Grech, V., Cox, J., & Caleja, N. (2007). Antenatal psychiatric moribidity in Maltese women. *General Hospital Psychiatry, 29*, 501-505.

Field, T., Diego, M., Dieter, J., Hernandez-Reif, M., Schanberg, S., Kuhn, C., . . . Bendell, D. (2004). Prenatal depression effects on the fetus and the newborn. *Infant Behavior and Development, 27*, 216-229.

Field, T., Diego, M., & Hernandez-Reif, M. (2006). Prenatal depression effects on the fetus and newborn: a review. *Infant Behav Dev, 29*(3), 445-455. 1934-8800 (Electronic) 0163-6383 (Linking).

Field, T., Diego, M., & Hernandez-Reif, M. (2010). Prenatal depression effects and interventions: a review. *Infant Behav Dev, 33*(4), 409-418. 1934-8800 (Electronic) 0163-6383 (Linking).

Field, T., Diego, M., Hernandez-Reif, M., Deeds, O., & Figueiredo, B. (2009). Pregnancy massage reduces prematurity, low birthweight and postpartum depression. *Infant Behav Dev, 32*(4), 454-460. 1934-8800 (Electronic) 0163-6383 (Linking).

Field, T., Diego, M., Hernandez-Reif, M., Figueiredo, B., Deeds, O., Ascencio, A., . . . Kuhn, C. (2010). Comorbid depression and anxiety effects on pregnancy and neonatal outcome. *Infant Behav Dev, 33*(1), 23-29. 1934-8800 (Electronic) 0163-6383 (Linking).

Field, T., Hernandez-Reif, M., & Diego, M. (2006). Newborns of depressed mothers who received moderate versus light pressure massage during pregnancy. *Infant Behav Dev, 29*(1), 54-58. 1934-8800 (Electronic) 0163-6383 (Linking).

Fink, N. S., Urech, C., Isabel, F., Meyer, A., Hoesli, I., Bitzer, J., & Alder, J. (2011). Fetal response to abbreviated relaxation techniques. A randomized controlled study. *Early Hum Dev, 87*(2), 121-127. 1872-6232 (Electronic) 0378-3782 (Linking).

Fisher, J. R., Tran, H. t. t., & Tran, T. (2007). Relative socioeconomic advantage and mood during advanced pregnancy in women in Vietnam. *International Journal of Mental Health Systems, 1*(3).

Flynn, H. A., Blow, F. C., & Marcus, S. M. (2006). Rates and predictors of depression treatment among pregnant women in hospital-affiliated obstetrics practices. *Gen Hosp Psychiatry, 28*(4), 289-295. 0163-8343 (Print) 0163-8343 (Linking).

Freeman, M. P. (2009). Complementary and alternative medicine for perinatal depression. *J Affect Disord, 112*(1-3), 1-10. 0165-0327 (Print) 0165-0327 (Linking).

Freeman, M. P., Davis, M., Sinha, P., Wisner, K. L., Hibbeln, J. R., & Gelenberg, A. J. (2008). Omega-3 fatty acids and supportive psychotherapy for perinatal depression: a randomized placebo-controlled study. *J Affect Disord, 110*(1-2), 142-148. 0165-0327 (Print) 0165-0327 (Linking).

Genesoni, L., & Tallandini, M. A. (2009). Men's psychological transition to fatherhood: an analysis of the literature, 1989-2008. *Birth, 36*(4), 305-318. 1523-536X (Electronic) 0730-7659 (Linking).

Gentile, S., & Galbally, M. (2011). Prenatal exposure to antidepressant medications and neurodevelopmental outcomes: a systematic review. *J Affect Disord, 128*(1-2), 1-9. 1573-2517 (Electronic) 0165-0327 (Linking).

Golbasi, Z., Kelleci, M., Kisacik, G., & Cetin, A. (2010). Prevalence and correlates of depression in pregnancy among Turkish women. *Maternal and Child Health journal, 14*, 485-491.

Grant, K.-A., McMahon, C., & Austin, M.-P. (2009). Maternal anxiety during the transition to parenthood: a prospective study. *Journal of Affective Disorders, 108*, 101-111.

Grant, K.-A., McMahon, C., Reilly, N., & Austin, M. P. (2010). Maternal sensitivity moderates the impact of prenatal anxiety disorder on infant responses to the still-face procedure. *Infant Behav Dev, 33*(4), 453-462. 1934-8800 (Electronic) 0163-6383 (Linking).

Grote, N. K., Bledsoe, S. E., Larkin, J., Lemay, E. P., & Brown, C. (2007). Stress exposure and depression in disadvantaged women: The protective effects of optimism and perceived control. *Social Work Research, 31*(1), 19-33. 1070-5309.

Grote, N. K., Swartz, H. A., Geibel, S. L., Zuckoff, A., Houck, P. R., & Frank, E. (2009). A randomized controlled trial of culturally relevant, brief interpersonal psychotherapy for perinatal depression. *Psychiatr Serv, 60*(3), 313-321. 1557-9700 (Electronic) 1075-2730 (Linking).

Halligan, S. L., Murray, L., Martins, C., & Cooper, P. J. (2007). Maternal depression and psychiatric outcomes in adolescent offspring: a 13-year longitudinal study. *J Affect Disord, 97*(1-3), 145-154. 0165-0327 (Print) 0165-0327 (Linking).

Harris, A., & Seckl, J. (2011). Glucocorticoids, prenatal stress and the programming of disease. *Horm Behav, 59*(3), 279-289. 1095-6867 (Electronic) 0018-506X (Linking).

Heron, J., O'Connor, T. G., Evans, J., Golding, J., & Glover, V. (2004). The course of anxiety and depression through pregnancy and the postpartum in a community sample. *J Affect Disord, 80*(1), 65-73. 0165-0327 (Print) 0165-0327 (Linking).

Heron, J., O'Connor, T. G., Evans, J., Golding, J., Glover, V., & Team, t. A. S. (2004). The course of anxiety and depression through pregnancy and the postpartum in a community sample. *Journal of Affective Disorders, 80*, 65-73.

Highet, N. J., Gemmill, A. W., & Milgrom, J. (2011). Depression in the perinatal period: awareness, attitudes and knowledge in the Australian population. *Australian and New Zealand Journal of Psychiatry, 45*, 223-231.

Ji, E. S., & Han, H. R. (2010). The effects of Qi exercise on maternal/fetal interaction and maternal well-being during pregnancy. *J Obstet Gynecol Neonatal Nurs, 39*(3), 310-318. 1552-6909 (Electronic) 0090-0311 (Linking).

Jomeen, J., & Martin, C. R. (2007). Replicability and stability of the multidimensional model of the Edinburgh Postnatal Depression Scale in late pregnancy. *J Psychiatr Ment Health Nurs, 14*(3), 319-324. 1351-0126 (Print) 1351-0126 (Linking).

Karmaliani, R., Asad, N., Bann, C. M., Moss, N., McClure, E. M., Pasha, O., . . . Goldenberg, R. L. (2009). Prevalence of anxiety, depression and associated factors among pregnant women of Hyderabad, Pakistan. *International Journal of Social Psychiatry, 55*(5), 414-424.

Kim, D. R., Sockol, L., Barber, J. P., Moseley, M., Lamprou, L., Rickels, K., . . . Epperson, C. N. (2011). A survey of patient acceptability of repetitive transcranial magnetic stimulation (TMS) during pregnancy. *J Affect Disord, 129*(1-3), 385-390. 1573-2517 (Electronic) 0165-0327 (Linking).

Kirpinar, I., Gozum, S., & Pasinlioglu, T. (2010). Prospective study of postpartum depression in eastern Turkey prevalence, socio-demographic and obstetric correlates, prenatal anxiety and early awareness. *J Clin Nurs, 19*(3-4), 422-431. 1365-2702 (Electronic) 0962-1067 (Linking).

Kopelman, R., & Stuart, S. (2005). Psychological treatments for postpartum depression. *Psychiatric Annals, 35*(7), 556-566. 0048-5713.

Lancaster, C. A., Gold, K. J., Flynn, H. A., Yoo, H., Marcus, S. M., & Davis, M. M. (2010). Risk factors for depressive symptoms during pregnancy: a systematic review. *Am J Obstet Gynecol, 202*(1), 5-14. 1097-6868 (Electronic) 0002-9378 (Linking).

Lara, M. A., Navarro, C., & Navarrete, L. (2010). Outcome results of a psycho-educational intervention in pregnancy to prevent PPD: A randomized control trial. *Journal of Affective Disorders, 122*(1-2), 109-117. 0165-0327.

Le, H. N., Perry, D. F., & Stuart, E. A. (2011). Randomized controlled trial of a preventive intervention for perinatal depression in high-risk Latinas. *J Consult Clin Psychol, 79*(2), 135-141. 1939-2117 (Electronic) 0022-006X (Linking).

Littleton, H. L., Bye, K., Buck, K., & Amacker, A. (2010). Psychosocial stress during pregnancy and perinatal outcomes: a meta-analytic review. *J Psychosom Obstet Gynaecol, 31*(4), 219-228. 1743-8942 (Electronic) 0167-482X (Linking).

Lobel, M., Cannella, D. L., Graham, J. E., DeVincent, C., Schneider, J., & Meyer, B. A. (2008). Pregnancy-specific stress, prenatal health behaviors, and birth outcomes. *Health Psychol, 27*(5), 604-615. 0278-6133 (Print) 0278-6133 (Linking).

Lox, C. L., & Treasure, D. C. (2000). Changes in feeling states following aquatic exercise during pregnancy. *Journal of Applied Social Psychology, 30*(3), 518-527. 0021-9029.

Manber, R., Schnyer, R. N., Allen, J. J., Rush, A. J., & Blasey, C. M. (2004). Acupuncture: a promising treatment for depression during pregnancy. *J Affect Disord, 83*(1), 89-95. 0165-0327 (Print) 0165-0327 (Linking).

Marcus, S. M. (2009). Depression during pregnancy: Rates, risks and consequences. *Canadian Journal of Clinical Pharmacology, 16*(1), e15-e22.

Mauri, M., oOppo, A., Montagnani, M. S., Borri, C., Banti, S., Camilleri, V., . . . Cassano, G. B. (2010). Beyond "postpartum depressions": specific anxiety diagnoses during pregnancy predict different outcomes. *Journal of Affective Disorders, 127*, 177-184.

Micali, N., Simonoff, E., & Treasure, J. (2011). Pregnancy and post-partum depression and anxiety in a longitudinal general population cohort: the effect of eating disorders and past depression. *Journal of Affective Disorders, 131*, 150-157.

Milgrom, J., Gemmill, A. W., Bilszta, J. L., Hayes, B., Barnett, B., Brooks, J., . . . Buist, A. (2008). Antenatal risk factors for postnatal depression: a large prospective study. *Journal of Affective Disorders, 108*, 147-157.

Milgrom, J., Schembri, C., Ericksen, J., Ross, J., & Gemmill, A. W. (2011). Towards parenthood: An antenatal intervention to reduce depression, anxiety and parenting difficulties. *Journal of Affective Disorders, 130*(3), 385-394. 0165-0327.

Miller, L., Shade, M., & Vasireddy, V. (2009). Beyond screening: assessment of perinatal depression in a perinatal care setting. *Arch Womens Ment Health, 12*(5), 329-334. 1435-1102 (Electronic).

Murray, L., & Cooper, P. J. (1997). Postpartum depression and child development. *Psychol Med, 27*(2), 253-260. 0033-2917 (Print) 0033-2917 (Linking).

Nasreen, H. E., Kabir, Z. N., Forsell, Y., & Edhborg, M. (2011). Prevalence and associated factors of depressive and anxiety symptoms during pregnancy: a population based study in rural Bangladesh. *BMC Womens Health, 11*, 22. 1472-6874 (Electronic) 1472-6874 (Linking).

Osmond, M., Wilkie, M., & Moore, J. (2002). *Behind the Smile: My Journey Out of Postpartum Depression* New York, NY: Grand Central Publishing.

Pottinger, A., Trotman-Edwards, H., & Younger, N. (2009). Detecting depression during pregnancy and associated lifestyle practices and concerns among women in a hospital-based obstetric clinic in Jamaica. *General Hospital Psychiatry, 31*, 254-261.

Poudevigne, M. S., & O'Connor, P. J. (2006). A review of physical activity patterns in pregnant women and their relationship to psychological health. *Sports Med, 36*(1), 19-38. 0112-1642 (Print) 0112-1642 (Linking).

Robertson, E., Grace, S., Wallington, T., & Stewart, D. E. (2004). Antenatal risk factors for postpartum depression: a synthesis of recent literature. *Gen Hosp Psychiatry, 26*(4), 289-295. 0163-8343 (Print) 0163-8343 (Linking).

Rogal, S. S., Poschman, K., Belanger, K., Howell, H. b., Smith, M. V., Medina, j., & Yonkers, K. A. (2007). Effects of postraumatic stress disorder on pregnancy outcomes. *Journal of Affective Disorders, 102*, 137-143.

Sawyer, A., Ayers, S., & Smith, H. (2010). Pre- and postnatal psychological wellbeing in Africa: a systematic review. *J Affect Disord, 123*(1-3), 17-29. 1573-2517 (Electronic) 0165-0327 (Linking).

Senturk, V., Abas, M., Berksun, O., & Stewart, R. (2011). Social support and antenatal depression in extended and nuclear family environments in Turkey: a cross-sectional survey. *BMC Psychiatry, 11*, 48.

Shields, B. (2005). *Down Came the Rain: My Journey Through Postpartum Depression* New York, NY: Hyperion.

Shivakumar, G., Brandon, A. R., Snell, P. G., Santiago-Munoz, P., Johnson, N. L., Trivedi, M. H., & Freeman, M. P. (2011). Antenatal depression: a rationale for studying exercise. *Depress Anxiety, 28*(3), 234-242. 1520-6394 (Electronic) 1091-4269 (Linking).

Smith, M. V., Shao, L., Howell, H., Wang, H., Poschman, K., & Yonkers, K. A. (2009). Success of mental health referral among pregnant and postpartum women with psychiatric distress. *Gen Hosp Psychiatry, 31*(2), 155-162. 1873-7714 (Electronic) 0163-8343 (Linking).

Sperlich, M., & Seng, J. (2008). *Survivor Moms: Women's Stories of Birthing, Mothering, and Healing after Sexual Abuse*. Eugene, Oregon: Motherbaby Press.

Spielberger, C. D., Gorsuch, R. L., Lushene, R., Vagg, P. R., & Jacobs, G. A. (1983). *Manual for the State-Trait Anxiety Inventory*. Palo Alto, CA: Consulting Psychologists Press Inc.

Spinelli, M. G., & Endicott, J. (2003). Controlled clinical trial of interpersonal psychotherapy versus parenting education program for depressed pregnant women. *Am J Psychiatry, 160*(3), 555-562. 0002-953X (Print) 0002-953X (Linking).

Swalm, D., Brooks, J., Doherty, D., Nathan, E., & Jacques, A. (2010). Using the Edinburgh postnatal depression scale to screen for perinatal anxiety. *Archives of Women's Mental Health, 13*, 515-522.

Teixeira, C., Figueiredo, B., Conde, A., Pacheco, A., & Costa, R. (2009). Anxiety and depression during pregnancy in women and men. *Journal of Affective Disorders, 119*, 142-148.

Uguz, F., Gezginc, K., Kayhan, F., Sarı, S., & Büyüköz, D. (2010). Is pregnancy associated with mood and anxiety disorders? A cross-sectional study. *General Hospital Psychiatry, 32*(2), 213-215.

Uguz, F., Gezginc, K., & Yazici, F. (2011). Are major depression and generalized anxiety disorder associated with intrauterine growth restriction in pregnant women? A case-control study. *Gen Hosp Psychiatry*. 1873-7714 (Electronic) 0163-8343 (Linking).

Urech, C., Fink, N. S., Hoesli, I., Wilhelm, F. H., Bitzer, J., & Alder, J. (2010). Effects of relaxation on psychobiological wellbeing during pregnancy: a randomized controlled trial. *Psychoneuroendocrinology, 35*(9), 1348-1355. 1873-3360 (Electronic) 0306-4530 (Linking).

van Bussel, J. C. H., Spitz, B., & Demyttenaere, K. (2006). Women's mental health before, during, and after pregnancy: a population-based controlled cohort study. *Birth, 33*(4), 297-302.

van Bussel, J. C. H., Spitz, B., & Demyttenaere, K. (2009). Anxiety in pregnant and postpartum women: an exploratory study of the role of maternal orientations. *Journal of Affective Disorders, 114*, 232-242.

Varma, D., Chandra, P. S., Thomas, T., & Carey, M. P. (2007). Intimate partner violence and sexual coercion among pregnant women in India: relationship with depression and post-traumatic stress disorder. *Journal of Affective Disorders, 102*, 227-235.

Whisman, M. A., Davila, J., & Goodman, S. H. (2011). Relationship adjustment, depression, and anxiety during pregnancy and the postpartum period. *J Fam Psychol, 25*(3), 375-383. 1939-1293 (Electronic) 0893-3200 (Linking).

Yonkers, K. A., Wisner, K. L., Stewart, D. E., Oberlander, T. F., Dell, D. L., Stotland, N., . . . Lockwood, C. (2009). The management of depression during pregnancy: a report from the American Psychiatric Association and the American College of Obstetricians and Gynecologists. *Gen Hosp Psychiatry, 31*(5), 403-413. 1873-7714 (Electronic) 0163-8343 (Linking).

3

# Perinatal Anxiety and Depression: Associations with Oxytocin and Mother-Infant Interactions

Rebecca McErlean and Valsamma Eapen
*University of New South Wales and Academic Unit of Child Psychiatry South West Sydney (AUCS)
Australia*

## 1. Introduction

There is converging evidence that heightened maternal anxiety and depression during the perinatal period affects early bonding and mother-infant interactions, exerting an important impact on the later development, competencies and mental health of the child. Yet there is a limited understanding of the biological mechanisms underpinning the link between perinatal mood and mother-infant interaction difficulties. This chapter will review the literature on the role of oxytocin in mediating bonding difficulties and infant outcome in women with perinatal anxiety and depression.

## 2. Maternal bonding and subsequent infant outcomes

The nature and quality of early parent-child relationships has been the subject of nearly a century of research stemming from attachment theory through to current biological approaches. Axiomatic to all approaches is the idea that successful human development is predicated on the establishment of a "bond". That is, the parent and child recognise, attend to and approach each other, are responsive to each other's states and communications, and experience feelings of 'closeness' and love (Brockington et al., 2001). All mammals are driven to seek predictable nurturing relationships with caregivers, and the successful negotiation of such early relationships lay the foundation for reaching maximum potentials in cognitive and social competence, and physical health (Meaney, 2001; Suomi, 1997). Large epidemiological studies show that early exposure to dysfunctional parenting is the single most significant (known) risk factor for childhood and later-onset mental disorders including depression, anxiety, disruptive behaviour, and substance abuse disorders (Green et al., 2010).

Both child and parent factors contribute to and derive benefits from, the successful establishment of such bonds. There is some evidence that the more sensitively the parent responds to their infant's cues the greater the likelihood that the infant will become securely attached (Atkinson et al., 2005; Bakermans-Kranenburg, van Ijzendoorn, & Juffer, 2003; De Wolff & van Ijzendoorn, 1997; Pederson, Gleason, Moran, & Bento, 1998; Seifer, Schiller, Sameroff, Resnick, & Riordan, 1996). Much of this research is based upon a classification system developed by Ainsworth that paid particular attention to the reaction of infants following a stressful situation (Ainsworth, 1979; Ainsworth, Blehar, Waters, & Wall, 1978). Attachment classifications are accorded in relation to the strength to which an infant uses their primary caregiver as a secure base, and also how avoidant or resistant the infant is when they resume contact with their mother after spending time with a stranger (see Ainsworth, et al., 1978; for full procedure). Secure attachment styles generally develop following positive maternal bonding experiences, including responsive and sensitive parenting. Once established, this style remains relatively consistent across the lifespan and if secure, will generally protect children from developing psychopathology such as anxiety, depression and aggression (Shaw, Owens, Giovannelli, & Winslow, 2001; Urban, Carlson, Egeland, & Sroufe, 1991; Warren, Huston, Egeland, & Sroufe, 1997); as well as enhancing their social competence and emotional regulation later in life (Elicker, Englund, Sroufe, Parke, & Ladd, 1992; Sroufe, 2005). The reverse is also the case with a meta-analysis revealing a significant association between an insecure maternal attachment in early childhood and later externalizing problems in children (Fearon & Belsky, 2011). Thus, improving maternal attachment and bonding within this early period can alter the trajectory of development towards more resilience in childhood and reduce the risk of developing mental health problems.

## 3. A role for oxytocin in maternal bonding

The biological basis of the "attachment-caregiving system" is slowly being elucidated with oxytocin continually being identified as the key component (Insel, 1997; Taylor et al., 2000). Oxytocin, as a neurohypophyseal hormone, is involved in the control of labour and secretion of milk via interaction with its receptors located in the uterus, mammary glands and peripheral tissues (Russell & Leng, 1998). Central oxytocin on the other hand has a key role in establishing and maintaining social affiliative behaviours (Lim & Young, 2006). The social affiliative properties of oxytocin are conserved across mammalian species (Keverne & Curley, 2004) along with the neural network of the oxytocinergic system (Tost et al., 2010) whereby oxytocin is produced within the Para ventricular nucleus and projects to limbic sites including the amygdala, ventral striatum, hypothalamus, nucleus accumbens and the mid brain (Sofroniew, 1983). Oxytocin facilitates the motivation to approach and engage others; it increases attention to, and the accurate perception of, salient social information; as well as improving social recognition. These are all essential processes in the formation of attachment bonds (Insel & Young, 2001). Conversely, there is emerging evidence that disruptions in oxytocin function are associated with impairments in social functioning and affiliative behaviours, including maternal bonding (Heinrichs & Gaab, 2007; Meyer-Lindenberg, Domes, Kirsch & Heinrichs, 2011). Given its well-researched, central role in initiating and maintaining successful bonding behaviours in non-human mammals (Insel, Krasnegor, & Bridges, 1990; Insel, Shapiro, Pedersen, Caldwell, & Jirikowski, 1992; Pedersen, Caldwell, Jirikowski, & Insel, 1992), oxytocin is proposed to also play an important role in the understanding and management of disrupted parent-child bonding in humans.

Baseline levels of peripherally measured plasma oxytocin are higher in women demonstrating positive bonding behaviours. Circulating plasma levels of oxytocin demonstrate high intra-individual stability throughout the pregnancy (Feldman, Weller, Zagoory-Sharon, & Levine, 2007; Gordon, Zagoory-Sharon, Leckman, & Feldman, 2010) and mothers whose levels peak around the birth report the greatest attachment to their unborn babies (Levine, Zagoory-Sharon, Feldman, & Weller, 2007). Around one month following the birth, these mothers demonstrate more maternal behaviours namely eye gaze, positive vocalisations, positive affect and affectionate touch. Moreover, mothers with higher levels of oxytocin also report more positive mental representations of their infants (Feldman, et al., 2007). Across the first six months of the infant's life both the levels of oxytocin and maternal behaviour are conserved, demonstrating a strong positive correlation at this time (Gordon, et al., 2010). Overall, plasma studies carried out in humans thus far mimic results from exhaustive investigations of the role of the neuropeptide in animals such as rats and voles with higher levels of oxytocin facilitatating species specific forms of maternal behaviour in the presence of infants.

## 4. Oxytocin as a mediator of the intergenerational transmission of attachment styles

Impairment in bonding not only affects the child's immediate psychological and cognitive development, it compromises neural functioning associated with future interpersonal relationships across the lifespan, including with one's own offspring. That is, poor relationship quality with a parent can irreversibly alter neuroanatomical structures in the brain that subsequently reduce the capacity for reinforcement value derived from interacting with one's own infants (Strathearn, Fonagy, Amico, & Montague, 2009; Swain, Lorberbaum, Kose, & Strathearn, 2007). Co-ordinated peripheral oxytocin release in the presence of infants alters as a function of maternal attachment style. Strathearn et al., (2009) found that only mothers with a secure attachment style demonstrated a peak in oxytocin levels during an interaction with their infants, measured when their infants were around seven months old. Mothers with an insecure attachment style showed a decrease in oxytocin levels during these interactive play sessions.

Thus, it seems that a mother's attachment style predicts her level of oxytocin release during interactions with her infant. More substantially, this oxytocin release co-occurs with periods of high levels of touch and affect-synchrony during play sessions, which directly influences her infant's concomitant release of oxytocin. Oxytocin levels in the mothers are mirrored by their infant's salivary oxytocin levels. The reactivity of both parties oxytocin system in response to one-to-one contact is also comparable, with the change scores from pre-post being significantly correlated (Feldman, Gordon, & Zagoory-Sharon, 2010). Furthermore, oxytocin levels are only increased in mothers who engage in high levels of affectionate touch during episodes of close infant contact (Feldman, Gordon, Schneiderman, Weisman, & Zagoory-Sharon, 2010) and increased oxytocin responsiveness is correlated with affect synchrony and infant social engagement (Feldman, Gordon, & Zagoory-Sharon, 2010). As physical touch in other contexts has been found to increase oxytocin levels, eg., during warm partner contact (Grewen, Girdler, Amico, & Light, 2005), 'affectionate touch' may be the necessary and sufficient transmitter of oxytocin levels between mother and infant which influence the responsiveness of the infants' oxytocin system. Oxytocin plasma levels and their pattern of release are transferred to the infant who subsequently adopts a similarly high frequency affectionate touching style with their own offspring.

Although human parenting behaviour is arguably more complex than behaviour seen in non-human animals, this theory is supported by animal data which demonstrates that oxytocin mediates mother-infant bonding through the act of maternal grooming, a behaviour analogous to affectionate touch in humans (Francis, Young, Meaney, & Insel, 2002). Maternal behaviour of increased licking and grooming of pups is associated with increased oxytocin receptor expression in rats. This behaviour is associated with reduced anxiety and better care overall for rat pups, akin to maternal sensitivity in humans (Francis, Champagne, & Meaney, 2000). Furthermore, their offspring resemble them behaviourally and neurobiologically through similarly reduced stress reactivity, denser oxytocin receptor expression in their brains and higher rates of maternal licking and grooming when they rear offspring, compared to pups of low licking/grooming mothers (Champagne, Diorio, Sharma, & Meaney, 2001; Francis, Diorio, Liu, & Meaney, 1999).

Due to the ability to manipulate rearing experiences through cross-fostering studies, the research group were able to show conclusively that environmental factors, in this case parenting style, can alter oxytocin expression in the brain and the subsequent parenting style adopted by offspring. The above pattern was reversed when female pups that were bred to high licking and grooming mothers were raised by low licking and grooming mothers. These infants then displayed the lower oxytocin receptor binding expected of the low licking grooming pups and went on to use the new low licking grooming style with their offspring (Champagne, 2008). This sequence of studies nicely depicts in one species the ever more complex gene by environment interactional explanations required to sequence the development of psychopathology (Champagne, 2011). From these studies we understand that the underlying genetics and maternal environment each play a critical role in predicting which maternal style infants ultimately adopt when they become parents themselves.

Parenting styles in humans have likewise been linked to underlying genetic susceptibility with mothers carrying the less efficient variant of the oxytocin receptor gene demonstrating poorer sensitivity towards their toddlers; acting as a less supportive presence to their children during a problem-solving task (Bakermans-Kranenburg & van Ijzendoorn, 2008). With genetic makeup determining oxytocin expression and parenting style directly influencing oxytocin responsiveness we can argue for a similarly complex gene by environment interplay in humans which ultimately transfers both parenting bonding style and oxytocin receptor expression through levels of affectionate touching. During face to face engagement with one's own infant, mothers differentially respond to social contact dependent upon their reported attachment style with their own parents. At the level of behavioural engagement with the infant, it has been noted that mothers whose oxytocin levels increase during the play engage in affectionately touching and stroking their infants. This would suggest that there is a feedback loop with oxytocin increasing as a function of touch for both the mother and the baby. The proposed mechanism by which this behaviour may be maintained is positive reinforcement derived through activation of the ventral striatum; the interface between mesolimbic dopaminergic and oxytocin systems (Skuse & Gallagher, 2009). A four month follow up of mothers whose oxytocin spiked during play sessions revealed a stronger ventral striatum response to both happy and sad expressions on their infant's face, compared to mothers with insecure attachment styles whose oxytocin levels dipped during the play session. The authors suggested that activation of this reward centre in the brain renders all stimuli associated with one's own child more rewarding, invoking maternal responsiveness to the infant's needs for securely attached mothers. The regulation of the oxytocin system *in the presence of relevant social stimuli* is therefore important: It was only *in the presence* of their infants that differences were observed in oxytocin levels, as both groups of mothers displayed similar baseline oxytocin levels. Furthermore, it must be *relevant social stimuli* as no differences were seen across all mothers, in ventral striatum activation, when they viewed infants who were not their own (Strathearn, Li, Fonagy, & Montague, 2008).

## 5. Perinatal anxiety, maternal bonding and oxytocin

Approximately 5-12% of women suffer from clinically diagnosed anxiety around the birth of their child, although sub clinical levels of distress which impact women's experiences of parenting may affect as many as 20-25% of mothers (Lonstein, 2007). Heightened maternal anxiety directly affects early mother-infant interactions (Barnett & Parker, 1985; Kaitz, Maytal, Devor, Bergman, & Mankuta, 2010). Anxiety during the pregnancy itself has the potential to significantly alter parenting such that it remains the single biggest predictor of children's later behavioural and emotional problems and heavily influences the mental competencies of the child (O'Connor, Heron, & Glover, 2002; O'Connor, Heron, Golding, Beveridge, & Glover, 2002). Some mothers find it hard to bond and connect to their new baby, and such failure in the context of anxiety may have long-term effects on the infant (Barnett & Parker, 1986). In this regard, an investigation of parental rearing styles conducted in six European countries found that low parental care and maternal overprotection were linked to anxiety disorders in the offspring, across the countries studied (Heider et al., 2008). It may be through the mechanism of overprotection that transmission of anxiety from mother to child occurs, with higher rates of anxiety diagnoses in children whose mothers suffer from an anxiety disorder (Schreier, Wittchen, Hofler, & Lieb, 2008).

Anxiety experienced by children with regard to separation from central attachment figures is of particular relevance in theoretical models of the transmission of attachment styles across generations. Individuals with separation anxiety have extreme anxiety about separations, actual or imagined, from significant others, usually, but not always, attachment figures (Manicavasagar, Silove, Curtis, & Wagner, 2000; Silove, Manicavasagar, & Drobny, 2002). Childhood separation anxiety is a DSM classified disorder (American Psychiatric Association, 2000). Anxiety specifically focused upon bonding with attachment figures in childhood activates a mental model of separation anxiety resulting in insecure attachment patterns of behaviour practiced throughout their lifetime (Manicavasagar, Silove, Marnane, & Wagner, 2009). Hence, researchers have argued for the continuity of separation anxiety in to adulthood, namely 'Adult Separation Anxiety Disorder' (Manicavasagar, Silove & Wagner, 2000). It has been suggested that there is a potential interaction between such anxiety and attachment style, with mothers having insecure attachment representations reporting heightened levels of maternal separation anxiety (Lutz & Hock, 1995). Mothers who report secure forms of attachment and who demonstrate more sensitive behaviour towards their infants are less likely to have children who develop separation anxiety (Dallaire and Weinraub, 2005). Thus, outcomes for children are mediated by maternal sensitivity. Support for this assertion comes from a finding that mother's mental representations of the attachment relationship were predictive of both their own level of maternal responsiveness and their child's attachment security demonstrated in the strange situation procedure at 18 months (Fonagy, Steele, & Steele, 1991). Maternal anxiety therefore exerts influence over a variety of crucial cognitive and behavioural repertoires in the mother, affecting subsequent mother-infant interactions and infant outcomes.

A complex gene-environment interaction has been proposed in the pathogenesis and intergenerational transmission of anxiety disorders (Eapen et al., 2005; Manicavasagar et al., 2001; Silove et al., 1995), a relationship which may be mediated through specific neuroendocrine modulators, including oxytocin and the hypothalamic-pituitary-adrenal (HPA) axis (Lonstein et al., 2007). Separation anxiety disorder in humans has been linked to a polymorphism of the oxytocin receptor gene (Costa et al., 2009) and one study has shown lower circulating levels of plasma oxytocin in patients with co-morbid depression and anxiety (Scantamburlo, et al., 2007). However, the majority of research has been carried out in non-human animals and supports the role of oxytocin in attenuating stress responses (eg. Lim and Young, 2006). A negative correlation between the levels of oxytocin and cortisol is not consistently observed, leading to speculation of a more complex interaction between oxytocin and the HPA axis. Instead of supporting a linear relationship between oxytocin and cortisol levels, research thus far appears to support a 'dysregulation' of both systems which results in inter-individual variability in how these systems respond during periods of stress and social affiliation. In reaction to stressful situations, peripheral oxytocin is typically released to attenuate stress (Nishioka et al., 1998; Wotjak et al., 1998). Although the mechanism of action is not entirely clear, it is suggested that high central oxytocin activity is anxiolytic and that such anxiolytic effects may partly be mediated through oxytocin's ability to modulate the release of excitatory amino acids (Ebner et al., 2005), and GABA (Brussaard, Wossink, Lodder, & Kits, 2000). Intracerebral oxytocin release in response to anxiogenic stimuli depends on personal past experiences and the inherent responsiveness of the mother's HPA axis (Bosch et al., 2005). In this regard, oxytocin knock-out mice exhibit more anxious behaviours and they also demonstrate reductions in maternal care toward their offspring (Mantella, Vollmer, Li, & Amico, 2003; Pedersen, Vadlamudi, Boccia, & Amico, 2006). Thus, both a mothers' oxytocin profile and her HPA axis regulation are important factors in determining her level of stress and social approach behaviours which may be directly transmitted to the foetus during periods of high antenatal anxiety (Huizink, Mulder, & Buitelaar, 2004).

We have seen that maternal attachment style predicts the responsiveness of the oxytocin system in the presence of infants, providing support for oxytocin facilitating positive social engagement and increasing the reward from the interaction. However, oxytocin release may be triggered by the stress of the situation and be acting as an anxiolytic (Uvnäs-Moberg, 1998). At this stage enough is not known about the direction of action between oxytocin and the HPA axis (Bicknell, 2003). Women with the highest rates of trait anxiety who may be the most likely to benefit from the anxiolytic effects of continual infant contact, are the least likely to initiate and persist in infant contact, including breastfeeding (Clifford, Campbell, Speechley, & Gorodzinsky, 2006; Forster et al., 2006; Papinczak & Turner, 2000). The lack of breastfeeding reduces the release of oxytocin by their infants suckling (Matthiesen, Ransjö-Arvidson, Nissen, & Uvnäs-Moberg, 2001) and as a lack of breast feeding is associated with decreased levels of oxytocin (Grewen, Davenport, & Light, 2010; Light et al., 2000; Mezzacappa & Endicott, 2007) these mothers would not be receiving the beneficial anxiolytic effects from breastfeeding. However, there is limited and inconclusive evidence in humans that physical contact with infants, even without breastfeeding, is an important contributor to positive mood and reduced anxiety in mothers (Lonstein, 2007).

## 6. Perinatal depression, maternal bonding and oxytocin

Between 10-20% of mothers suffer from perinatal depression (O'Hara & Swain, 1996) and many more experience subclinical levels of depression around the birth of their child. When identified risk factors for depression are controlled for, women who have given birth are 1.6 times more likely to develop depression as compared to women who have not had children (Eberhard-Gran, Eskild, Tambs, Samuelsen, & Opjordsmoen, 2002). Regarding the aetiology of depression in the postpartum period, similar risk factors to other episodes of depression have been identified, including: a past history of depression; previous treatment for emotional problems; a poor relationship with the partner; and experiencing a large number of negative life events in the previous 12 months (Eberhard-Gran, et al., 2002; Leigh & Milgrom, 2008; Milgrom et al., 2008; Whiffen & Gotlib, 1993). However, primiparity and antenatal anxiety are risk factors unique to postnatal depression, independent of previous episodes of depression (Eberhard-Gran, et al., 2002; Leigh & Milgrom, 2008). Twenty-nine per cent of women who experience antenatal depression also report significant depressive symptoms in the postpartum period (Milgrom, et al., 2008). Furthermore, mothers who report excessive anxiety or worry during the antenatal period are more likely to report postnatal depression (Austin, Tully, & Parker, 2007). Cooper and colleagues (2007) failed to find significant phenomenological differences in the clinical symptom presentation for three groups of women who were all suffering from recurrent episodes of clinical depression: those who were currently suffering from postnatal depression; those who had suffered from an episode of postnatal depression; or mothers who were suffering recurrent episodes of depression but had not had an episode following the birth of their child/ren (Cooper et al., 2007). Some minor differences were noted in that postnatally depressed women were less likely to report poor appetite, morning wakening and slowed activity. However, the authors noted that this could be explained by a general increase in appetite during breastfeeding, generally disrupted sleep after the child's birth and increased activities relating to childrearing. Mixed results for symptom course and duration are reported with some studies finding a longer duration for depressive episodes following the birth of a child whilst others reporting that depressive episodes across their sample had a similar pattern of remission within a six-month period (Cooper, et al., 2007; Kumar & Robson, 1984; Whiffen & Gotlib, 1993). Whiffen and Gotlib (1993) also observed that episodes of postnatal depression are generally milder than other episodes of depression.

Therefore, for the most part, postnatal depression closely resembles other episodes of depression. The most noteworthy difference is that the psychiatric disturbance occurs at a critical period in the infant's development, which singles out maternal postnatal depression as a worthwhile enterprise for research attention. Depression experienced by a parent at any time impacts on a child's development, however it is even more potent at this early stage in development when an infant is acquiring the basic skills required for all subsequent language, cognitive, behavioural, social and emotional development. Postnatal depression has been found to have adverse consequences across multiple domains of the mother's life. Higher levels of postnatal depression have been associated with reduced maternal sleep

(Meltzer & Mindell, 2007) and increased parental stress (Milgrom & McCloud, 1996). Depressed mothers do not experience the joys and challenges of parenting in the same way as non-depressed mothers; reporting lower levels of competence, poorer emotional attachment to their infant, poorer health and more restricted and more socially isolated feelings than non-depressed mothers. Furthermore, they were more likely to report poorer marital quality, higher tension, confusion, anger, fatigue and lower levels of vigour than non-depressed mothers (Milgrom & McCloud, 1996). Although self-reported depression decreased over the study period of 3-12 months, negative ratings of their relationship with their child and their spouse were maintained.

Mothers who suffer from postnatal depression also interact differently with their infants. This has been well documented in numerous studies comparing the behaviour of depressed and non-depressed women. They demonstrate less sensitive, less affirming and more negating behaviours towards their infants (Murray, Fiori-Cowley, Hooper, & Cooper, 1996) and are more likely to show increased negative affect, less imitation and game playing, and less contingent responses (Field et al., 1985). Affectionate contact is also reduced and there are less vocalisations and responses to the infant's vocalisations (Fleming, Ruble, Flett, & Shaul, 1988). On the whole, they demonstrate less sensitive responding to their infant's cues (Cox, Puckering, Pound, & Mills, 1987). Evidence exists for mother's negative attitudinal and behavioural repertoires noticeably altering infant's behaviour over the short and long term. Infants of postnatally depressed mothers show less engagement (Murray, Fiori-Cowley, et al., 1996), they are drowsier and fussier, and they appear less relaxed and show less content expressions (Field, et al., 1985) when observed during early interactions with their mothers. Their performance on object concept tasks are impaired at 12 months (Murray, 1992) and this finding has been supported by other follow up studies which observed these infants to be suffering from cognitive developmental delays compared to their age matched peers (Lyons-Ruth, Zoll, Connell, & Grunebaum, 1986; Murray, Fiori-Cowley, et al., 1996). When infants were assessed at 19 months, those with a mother who had suffered from postnatal depression during their first year were found to be angrier, they showed less affectionate sharing and were less sociable with strangers (Stein et al., 1991). These children were also more at risk for developing emotional and behavioural problems during early childhood (Billings & Moos, 1983; Lynne, 1992; Murray, 1992; Murray, Hipwell, Hooper, Stein, & Cooper, 1996).

The negative observed outcomes at 18-19 months were also demonstrated in infants whose mother's depression remitted within three to six months (Murray, 1992; Stein, et al., 1991), indicating that it is the changed interaction style established between a mother and her infant during this time, which persists beyond the depressive episode, that is responsible for influencing infant outcomes. A five year follow up of children of depressed mothers supported this theory with maternal insensitivity predicting poorer outcomes for children, independently of the mothers' level of depression (Murray, Hipwell, et al., 1996). Mothers suffering from depression are also at an increased risk of developing bonding difficulties. A third of women with postnatal depression will report bonding problems with their infants, and even mild levels of depression are associated with increased bonding difficulties (Brockington, et al., 2001; Moehler, Brunner, Wiebel, Reck, & Resch, 2006). A subsample of these women will report severe rejection of, and anger toward, their infant (Loh & Vostanis, 2004).

Children whose mothers experience bonding difficulties and respond less sensitively to them aren't as securely attached to their mothers around two years of age (Bakermans-Kranenburg, et al., 2003). In addition, exposure to maternal depression early in life is an independent significant predictor of poorer attachment (Martins & Gaffan, 2000). All of the researchers who have investigated this relationship have concluded that depression in the mother has significant adverse outcomes on the infant's attachment to her and therefore results in less secure forms of attachment as measured by the strange situation procedure, or a variant thereof (Lyons-Ruth, et al., 1986; Murray, Fiori-Cowley, et al., 1996; Radke-Yarrow, Cummings, Kuczynski, & Chapman, 1985; Teti, Gelfand, Messinger, & Isabella, 1995)..

The link between oxytocin and depressive symptoms has not been illuminated with research returning either null findings or a positive correlation between the two (Scantamburlo et al., 2007; van Londen et al., 1997). Researchers have speculated upon a link with oxytocin as it has direct effects upon the HPA axis, the dysregulation of which is heavily implicated in major depressive disorder (Pariante & Lightman, 2008). Cyranowski et al., (2008) found that depressed women did not display the same pattern of oxytocin release during emotional and stress inducing tasks, arguing for the dysregulation of oxytocin release in these women. Recent evidence supporting a negative correlation between oxytocin and depressive symptoms has emerged from a study directly investigating women's oxytocin levels during late pregnancy. Skrundz and colleagues (Skrundz, Bolten, Nast, Hellhammer, & Meinlschmidt, 2011) found that in approximately 8/10 cases they were accurately able to predict a women's risk of developing postnatal depressive symptoms at two weeks postpartum from an analysis of her oxytocin levels. Women with lower levels of oxytocin were susceptible to low mood in the early postpartum. Some of these women are prone to developing bonding difficulties with their infant and this data ties in with Feldman's results of decreased oxytocin levels being associated with poorer bonding behaviours around this time (Feldman, 2007; Feldman, et al., 2007).

This relationship is further complicated by breastfeeding status in these women as we have seen that oxytocin levels increase during feeding and depressed mothers cease breastfeeding earlier than mothers who have not suffered from postnatal depression. Ninety-three percent of these women report ceasing breastfeeding at the time of, or after the onset of postnatal depression (Henderson, Evans, Straton, Priest, & Hagan, 2003). Additionally, mothers who are not breastfeeding report higher levels of postnatal depression than those who do breastfeed (Eberhard-Gran, et al., 2002). Therefore, mothers with depression may not be receiving the beneficial effects of increased oxytocin (Grewen, et al., 2010; Matthiesen, et al., 2001), and it may be that this is due to a neurobiological deficit in naturally circulating levels of oxytocin which acts as a risk factor for both postnatal depression and breastfeeding difficulties. This remains speculative as longitudinal research is yet to be carried out within this population.

## 7. Conclusion

It is plausible that mothers with anxiety and depression mediated through low levels of oxytocin would be particularly vulnerable to negative mother-infant interactions as they find the interactions with their child less rewarding or more anxiety provoking. These patterns may set the stage for the development of psychopathology in the developing child leading to adverse mental health outcomes in adulthood. Affected adults in turn will have attachment difficulties in rearing their own infants creating a transmission of parenting styles across generations. The investigation of oxytocin in human maternal affiliation and separation behaviours is in its early stages. However there is emerging evidence to implicate oxytocin in patterns of maternal bonding, with higher oxytocin levels in mothers with secure attachment rendering stimuli associated with their own child more rewarding, thereby facilitating maternal sensitivity and responsiveness and improving the quality of bonding and attachment with the infant. Nevertheless, the role of maternal mood in this process is less clear and further studies examining relevant neurobiological parameters, especially the association of maternal anxiety, depression and attachment behaviours with oxytocin, and other indices of hypothalamic-pituitary-adrenal axis functioning, are indicated. Such research would open up the possibility of early psychological interventions and pharmacological therapies targeting oxytocin and the HPA axis that would improve maternal mood and prevent the development of potentially maladaptive mother-infant interactions resulting in better maternal and infant outcomes.

## 8. References

Ainsworth, M. S. (1979). Infant-mother attachment. *American Psychologist, 34*(10), 932-937. doi: 10.1037/0003-066x.34.10.932

Ainsworth, M. S., Blehar, M. C., Waters, E., & Wall, S. (1978). *Patterns of attachment: A psychological study of the strange situation*: Lawrence Erlbaum: Oxford.

American Psychiatric Association. Task Force on, D.-I. (2000). *Diagnostic and statistical manual of mental disorders : DSM-IV-TR*. Washington, DC: American Psychiatric Association.

Atkinson, L., Goldberg, S., Raval, V., Pederson, D., Benoit, D., Moran, G., . . . Leung, E. (2005). On the Relation Between Maternal State of Mind and Sensitivity in the Prediction of Infant Attachment Security. *Developmental Psychology, 41*(1), 42-53. doi: 10.1037/0012-1649.41.1.42

Austin, M.-P., Tully, L., & Parker, G. (2007). Examining the relationship between antenatal anxiety and postnatal depression. *Journal of Affective Disorders, 101*(1-3), 169-174. doi: 10.1016/j.jad.2006.11.015

Bakermans-Kranenburg, M. J., & van Ijzendoorn, M. H. (2008). Oxytocin receptor (OXTR) and serotonin transporter (5-HTT) genes associated with observed parenting. *Soc Cogn Affect Neurosci, 3*(2), 128-134. doi: 10.1093/scan/nsn004

Bakermans-Kranenburg, M. J., van Ijzendoorn, M. H., & Juffer, F. (2003). Less is more: Meta-analyses of sensitivity and attachment interventions in early childhood. *Psychological Bulletin, 129*(2), 195-215.

Barnett, B., & Parker, G. (1985). Professional and non-professional intervention for highly anxious primiparous mothers. *The British Journal of Psychiatry, 146*(3), 287-293. doi: 10.1192/bjp.146.3.287

Bicknell, J. (2003). Depression, Stress and the Adrenal axis. *Journal of Neuroendocrinology, 15*(8), 811-812. doi: 10.1046/j.1365-2826.2003.01058.x

Billings, A. G., & Moos, R. H. (1983). Comparisons of children of depressed and nondepressed parents: A social-environmental perspective. *Journal of Abnormal Child Psychology, 11*(4), 463-485. doi: 10.1007/bf00917076

Brockington, I. F., Oates, J., George, S., Turner, D., Vostanis, P., Sullivan, M., . . . Murdoch, C. (2001). A Screening Questionnaire for mother-infant bonding disorders. *Archives of Women's Mental Health, 3*(4), 133-140.

Brussaard, A. B., Wossink, J., Lodder, J. C., & Kits, K. S. (2000). Progesterone-metabolite prevents protein kinase C-dependent modulation of Î³-aminobutyric acid type A receptors in oxytocin neurons. *Proceedings of the National Academy of Sciences of the United States of America, 97*(7), 3625-3630.

Champagne, F. A. (2008). Epigenetic mechanisms and the transgenerational effects of maternal care. *Frontiers in Neuroendocrinology, 29*(3), 386-397.

Champagne, F. A. (2011). Maternal imprints and the origins of variation. *Hormones and Behavior,* No Pagination Specified. doi: 10.1016/j.yhbeh.2011.02.016

Champagne, F. A., Diorio, J., Sharma, S., & Meaney, M. J. (2001). Naturally occurring variations in maternal behavior in the rat are associated with differences in estrogen-inducible central oxytocin receptors. *Proceedings of the National Academy of Sciences of the United States of America, 98*(22), 12736-12741.

Clifford, T. J., Campbell, M. K., Speechley, K. N., & Gorodzinsky, F. (2006). Factors Influencing Full Breastfeeding in a Southwestern Ontario Community: Assessments at 1 Week and at 6 Months Postpartum. *Journal of Human Lactation, 22*(3), 292-304. doi: 10.1177/0890334406290043

Cooper, C., Jones, L., Dunn, E., Forty, L., Haque, S., Oyebode, F., . . . Jones, I. (2007). Clinical presentation of postnatal and non-postnatal depressive episodes. *Psychological Medicine, 37*(9), 1273-1280. doi: 10.1017/s0033291707000116

Cox, A., Puckering, C., Pound, A., & Mills, M. (1987). The impact of maternal depression in young children. *Journal of Child Psychology and Psychiatry, 28*(6), 917-928. doi: 10.1111/j.1469-7610.1987.tb00679.x

Cyranowski, J. M., Hofkens, T. L., Frank, E., Seltman, H., Cai, H.-M., & Amico, J. A. (2008). Evidence of dysregulated peripheral oxytocin release among depressed women. *Psychosomatic Medicine, 70*(9), 967-975. doi: 10.1097/PSY.0b013e318188ade4

De Wolff, M. S., & van Ijzendoorn, M. H. (1997). Sensitivity and Attachment: A Meta-Analysis on Parental Antecedents of Infant Attachment. *Child Development, 68*(4), 571-591. doi: 10.1111/j.1467-8624.1997.tb04218.x

Eberhard-Gran, M., Eskild, A., Tambs, K., Samuelsen, S. O., & Opjordsmoen, S. (2002). Depression in postpartum and non-postpartum women: prevalence and risk factors. *Acta Psychiatrica Scandinavica, 106*(6), 426-433.

Elicker, J., Englund, M., Sroufe, L. A., Parke, R. D., & Ladd, G. W. (1992). Predicting peer competence and peer relationships in childhood from early parent-child relationships *Family-peer relationships: Modes of linkage.* (pp. 77-106): Lawrence Erlbaum Associates.

Fearon, P. R. M., & Belsky, J. (2011). Infant–mother attachment and the growth of externalizing problems across the primary-school years. *Journal of Child Psychology and Psychiatry,* no-no. doi: 10.1111/j.1469-7610.2010.02350.x

Feldman, R. (2007). Parent-Infant Synchrony: Biological Foundations and Developmental Outcomes. *Current Directions in Psychological Science, 16*(6), 340-345. doi: doi:10.1111/j.1467-8721.2007.00532.x

Feldman, R., Gordon, I., Schneiderman, I., Weisman, O., & Zagoory-Sharon, O. (2010). Natural variations in maternal and paternal care are associated with systematic changes in oxytocin following parent-infant contact. *Psychoneuroendocrinology, 35,* 1133-1141.

Feldman, R., Gordon, I., & Zagoory-Sharon, O. (2010). The cross-generation transmission of oxytocin in humans. *Hormones and Behavior, 58*(4), 669-676. doi: DOI: 10.1016/j.yhbeh.2010.06.005

Feldman, R., Weller, A., Zagoory-Sharon, O., & Levine, A. (2007). Evidence for a neuroendocrinological foundation of human affiliation: Plasma oxytocin levels across pregnancy and the postpartum period predict mother-infant bonding. *Psychological Science, 18*(11), 965-970.

Field, T., Sandberg, D., Garcia, R., Vega-Lahr, N., Goldstein, S., & Guy, L. (1985). Pregnancy problems, postpartum depression, and early mother-infant interactions. *Developmental Psychology, 21*(6), 1152-1156. doi: 10.1037/0012-1649.21.6.1152

Fleming, A. S., Ruble, D. N., Flett, G. L., & Shaul, D. L. (1988). Postpartum adjustment in first-time mothers: Relations between mood, maternal attitudes, and mother-infant interactions. *Developmental Psychology, 24*(1), 71-81. doi: 10.1037/0012-1649.24.1.71

Fonagy, P., Steele, H., & Steele, M. (1991). Maternal representations of attachment during pregnancy predict the organization of infant-mother attachment at one year of age. *Child Development, 62*(5), 891-905. doi: 10.2307/1131141

Francis D. D., Diorio, J., Liu, D., & Meaney, M. J. (1999). Nongenomic Transmission Across Generations of Maternal Behavior and Stress Responses in the Rat. *Science, 286*(5442), 1155-1158. doi: 10.1126/science.286.5442.1155

Francis, D. D., Champagne, F. C., & Meaney, M. J. (2000). Variations in Maternal Behaviour are Associated with Differences in Oxytocin Receptor Levels in the Rat. *Journal of Neuroendocrinology, 12*(12), 1145-1148. doi: 10.1046/j.1365-2826.2000.00599.x

Francis, D. D., Young, L. J., Meaney, M. J., & Insel, T. R. (2002). Naturally Occurring Differences in Maternal Care are Associated with the Expression of Oxytocin and Vasopressin (V1a) Receptors: Gender Differences. *Journal of Neuroendocrinology, 14*(5), 349-353.

Gordon, I., Zagoory-Sharon, O., Leckman, J. F., & Feldman, R. (2010). Oxytocin, cortisol, and triadic family interactions. *Physiology & Behavior, 101*(5), 679-684.

Green, J. G., McLaughlin, K. A., Berglund, P. A., Gruber, M. J., Sampson, N. A., Zaslavsky, A. M., & Kessler, R. C. (2010). Childhood Adversities and Adult Psychiatric Disorders in the National Comorbidity Survey Replication I: Associations With First Onset of DSM-IV Disorders. *Arch Gen Psychiatry, 67*(2), 113-123. doi: 10.1001/archgenpsychiatry.2009.186

Grewen, K. M., Davenport, R. E., & Light, K. C. (2010). An investigation of plasma and salivary oxytocin responses in breast- and formula-feeding mothers of infants. *Psychophysiology, 47*(4), 625-632. doi: 10.1111/j.1469-8986.2009.00968.x

Grewen, K. M., Girdler, S. S., Amico, J., & Light, K. C. (2005). Effects of Partner Support on Resting Oxytocin, Cortisol, Norepinephrine, and Blood Pressure Before and After Warm Partner Contact. *Psychosomatic Medicine, 67*(4), 531-538. doi: 10.1097/01.psy.0000170341.88395.47

Heinrichs, M., & Gaab, J. (2007). Neuroendocrine mechanisms of stress and social interaction: Implications for mental disorders. *Current Opinion in Psychiatry, 20*(2), 158-162. doi: 10.1097/YCO.0b013e3280146a13

Henderson, J. J., Evans, S. F., Straton, J. A. Y., Priest, S. R., & Hagan, R. (2003). Impact of postnatal depression on breastfeeding duration. *Birth: Issues in Perinatal Care, 30*(3), 175-180. doi: 10.1046/j.1523-536X.2003.00242.x

Insel, T. R. (1997). A neurobiological basis of social attachment. *American Journal of Psychiatry, 154*(6), 726-735.

Insel, T. R., Krasnegor, N. A., & Bridges, R. S. (1990). Oxytocin and maternal behavior *Mammalian parenting: Biochemical, neurobiological, and behavioral determinants.* (pp. 260-280): Oxford University Press: New York.

Insel, T. R., Shapiro, L. E., Pedersen, C. A., Caldwell, J. D., & Jirikowski, G. F. (1992). Oxytocin receptors and maternal behavior *Oxytocin in maternal, sexual, and social behaviors.* (pp. 122-141): New York Academy of Sciences: New York.

Insel, T. R., & Young, L. J. (2001). The neurobiology of attachment. *Nat Rev Neurosci, 2*(2), 129-136.

Kaitz, M., Maytal, H. R., Devor, N., Bergman, L., & Mankuta, D. (2010). Maternal anxiety, mother–infant interactions, and infants' response to challenge. *Infant Behavior & Development, 33*(2), 136-148. doi: 10.1016/j.infbeh.2009.12.003

Keverne, E. B., & Curley, J. P. (2004). Vasopressin, oxytocin and social behaviour. *Current Opinion in Neurobiology, 14*(6), 777-783. doi: DOI: 10.1016/j.conb.2004.10.006

Kumar, R., & Robson, K. M. (1984). A prospective study of emotional disorders in childbearing women. *British Journal of Psychiatry, 144*, 35-47.

Leigh, B., & Milgrom, J. (2008). Risk factors for antenatal depression, postnatal depression and parenting stress. *BMC Psychiatry, 8*(1), 24.

Levine, A., Zagoory-Sharon, O., Feldman, R., & Weller, A. (2007). Oxytocin during pregnancy and early postpartum: Individual patterns and maternal-fetal attachment. *Peptides, 28*(6), 1162-1169.

Light, K. C., Smith, T. E., Johns, J. M., Brownley, K. A., Hofheimer, J. A., & Amico, J. A. (2000). Oxytocin responsivity in mothers of infants: A preliminary study of relationships with blood pressure during laboratory stress and normal ambulatory activity. *Health Psychology, 19*(6), 560-567. doi: 10.1037/0278-6133.19.6.560

Lim, M. M., & Young, L. J. (2006). Neuropeptidergic regulation of affiliative behavior and social bonding in animals. *Hormones and Behavior, 50*(4), 506-517. doi: 10.1016/j.yhbeh.2006.06.028

Loh, C.-C., & Vostanis, P. (2004). Perceived mother-infant relationship difficulties in postnatal depression. *Infant and Child Development, 13*(2), 159-171. doi: 10.1002/icd.347

Lonstein, J. S. (2007). Regulation of anxiety during the postpartum period. *Frontiers in Neuroendocrinology, 28*(2-3), 115-141. doi: 10.1016/j.yfrne.2007.05.002

Lutz, W. J., & Hock, E. (1995). Maternal Separation Anxiety: Relations to Adult Attachment Representations in Mothers of Infants. *The Journal of Genetic Psychology: Research and Theory on Human Development, 156*(1), 57 - 72.

Lynne, M. (1992). The Impact of Postnatal Depression on Infant Development. *Journal of Child Psychology and Psychiatry, 33*(3), 543-561.

Lyons-Ruth, K., Zoll, D., Connell, D., & Grunebaum, H. U. (1986). The depressed mother and her one-year-old infant: Environment, interaction, attachment, and infant development. *New Directions for Child Development, 34*, 61-82.

Manicavasagar, V., Silove, D., Curtis, J., & Wagner, R. (2000). Continuities of separation anxiety from early life into adulthood. *Journal of Anxiety Disorders, 14*(1), 1-18. doi: 10.1016/s0887-6185(99)00029-8

Mantella, R. C., Vollmer, R. R., Li, X., & Amico, J. A. (2003). Female Oxytocin-Deficient Mice Display Enhanced Anxiety-Related Behavior. *Endocrinology, 144*(6), 2291-2296. doi: 10.1210/en.2002-0197

Martins, C., & Gaffan, E. A. (2000). Effects of early maternal depression on patterns of infant-mother attachment: A meta-analytic investigation. *Journal of Child Psychology and Psychiatry, 41*(6), 737-746.

Matthiesen, A.-S., Ransjö-Arvidson, A.-B., Nissen, E., & Uvnäs-Moberg, K. (2001). Postpartum maternal oxytocin release by newborns: Effects of infant hand massage and sucking. *Birth: Issues in Perinatal Care, 28*(1), 13-19. doi: 10.1046/j.1523-536X.2001.00013.x

Meyer-Lindenberg, A., Domes, G., Kirsch, P., & Heinrichs, M. (2011). Oxytocin and vasopressin in the human brain: social neuropeptides for translational medicine. [10.1038/nrn3044]. *Nat Rev Neurosci, 12*(9), 524-538. doi: http://www.nature.com/nrn/journal/v12/n9/suppinfo/nrn3044_S1.html

Meaney, M. J. (2001). Maternal care, gene expression, and the transmission of individual differences in stress reactivity across generations. *Annual Review of Neuroscience, 24*(1), 1161-1192. doi: doi:10.1146/annurev.neuro.24.1.1161

Meltzer, L. J., & Mindell, J. A. (2007). Relationship between child sleep disturbances and maternal sleep, mood, and parenting stress: A pilot study. *Journal of Family Psychology, 21*(1), 67-73. doi: 10.1037/0893-3200.21.1.67

Mezzacappa, E. S., & Endicott, J. (2007). Parity mediates the association between infant feeding method and maternal depressive symptoms in the postpartum. *Archives of Women's Mental Health, 10*(6), 259-266.

Milgrom, J., Gemmill, A. W., Bilszta, J. L., Hayes, B., Barnett, B., Brooks, J., . . . Buist, A. (2008). Antenatal risk factors for postnatal depression: A large prospective study. *Journal of Affective Disorders, 108*(1-2), 147-157.

Milgrom, J., & McCloud, P. I. (1996). Parenting stress and postnatal depression. *Stress Medicine, 12*(3), 177 - 186.

Moehler, E., Brunner, R., Wiebel, A., Reck, C., & Resch, F. (2006). Maternal depressive symptoms in the postnatal period are associated with long-term impairment of mother-child bonding. *Archives of Women's Mental Health, 9*(5), 273-278. doi: 10.1007/s00737-006-0149-5

Murray, L. (1992). The impact of postnatal depression on infant development. *Journal of Child Psychology and Psychiatry, 33*(3), 543-561. doi: 10.1111/j.1469-7610.1992.tb00890.x

Murray, L., Fiori-Cowley, A., Hooper, R., & Cooper, P. (1996). The impact of postnatal depression and associated adversity on early mother-infant interactions and later infant outcomes. *Child Development, 67*(5), 2512-2526. doi: 10.2307/1131637

Murray, L., Hipwell, A., Hooper, R., Stein, A., & Cooper, P. (1996). The Cognitive Development of 5-Year-Old Children of Postnatally Depressed Mothers. *Journal of Child Psychology and Psychiatry, 37*(8), 927-935.

O'Connor, T. G., Heron, J., & Glover, V. (2002). Antenatal anxiety predicts child behavioral/emotional problems independently of postnatal depression. *Journal of the American Academy of Child & Adolescent Psychiatry, 41*(12), 1470-1477. doi: 10.1097/00004583-200212000-00019

O'Connor, T. G., Heron, J., Golding, J., Beveridge, M., & Glover, V. (2002). Maternal antenatal anxiety and children's behavioural/emotional problems at 4 years: Report from the Avon Longitudinal Study of Parents and Children. *The British Journal of Psychiatry, 180*(6), 502-508. doi: 10.1192/bjp.180.6.502

O'Hara, M. W., & Swain, A. (1996). Rates and risk of postpartum depression - a meta-analysis. *International Review of Psychiatry, 8*, 37 - 54.

Papinczak, T. A., & Turner, C. T. (2000). An analysis of personal and social factors influencing initiation and duration of breastfeeding in a large Queensland maternity hospital. *Breastfeeding review : professional publication of the Nursing Mothers" Association of Australia, 8*(1), 25-33.

Pariante, C. M., & Lightman, S. L. (2008). The HPA axis in major depression: Classical theories and new developments. *Trends in Neurosciences, 31*(9), 464-468. doi: 10.1016/j.tins.2008.06.006

Pedersen, C. A., Caldwell, J. D., Jirikowski, G. F., & Insel, T. R. (1992). *Oxytocin in maternal, sexual, and social behaviors*: New York Academy of Sciences: New York.

Pedersen, C. A., Vadlamudi, S. V., Boccia, M. L., & Amico, J. A. (2006). Maternal behavior deficits in nulliparous oxytocin knockout mice. *Genes, Brain and Behavior, 5*(3), 274-281. doi: 10.1111/j.1601-183X.2005.00162.x

Pederson, D. R., Gleason, K. E., Moran, G., & Bento, S. (1998). Maternal attachment representations, maternal sensitivity, and the infant-mother attachment relationship. *Developmental Psychology, 34*(5), 925-933. doi: 10.1037/0012-1649.34.5.925

Radke-Yarrow, M., Cummings, E. M., Kuczynski, L., & Chapman, M. (1985). Patterns of attachment in two- and three-year-olds in normal families and families with parental depression. *Child Development, 56*(4), 884-893. doi: 10.2307/1130100

Russell, J. A., & Leng, G. (1998). Sex, parturition and motherhood without oxytocin? *J Endocrinol, 157*(3), 343-359. doi: 10.1677/joe.0.1570343

Scantamburlo, G., Hansenne, M., Fuchs, S., Pitchot, W., Maréchal, P., Pequeux, C., . . . Legros, J. J. (2007). Plasma oxytocin levels and anxiety in patients with major depression. *Psychoneuroendocrinology, 32*(4), 407-410.

Schreier, A., Wittchen, H.-U., Hofler, M., & Lieb, R. (2008). Anxiety disorders in mothers and their children: prospective longitudinal community study. *The British Journal of Psychiatry, 192*(4), 308-309. doi: 10.1192/bjp.bp.106.033589

Seifer, R., Schiller, M., Sameroff, A. J., Resnick, S., & Riordan, K. (1996). Attachment, maternal sensitivity, and infant temperament during the first year of life. *Developmental Psychology, 32*(1), 12-25. doi: 10.1037/0012-1649.32.1.12

Shaw, D. S., Owens, E. B., Giovannelli, J., & Winslow, E. B. (2001). Infant and toddler pathways leading to early externalizing disorders. *Journal of the American Academy of Child & Adolescent Psychiatry, 40*(1), 36-43. doi: 10.1097/00004583-200101000-00014

Silove, D., Manicavasagar, V., & Drobny, J. (2002). Associations between juvenile and adult forms of separation anxiety disorder: A study of volunteers with histories of school refusal. *Journal of Nervous and Mental Disease, 190*(6), 413-414. doi: 10.1097/00005053-200206000-00013

Skrundz, M., Bolten, M., Nast, I., Hellhammer, D. H., & Meinlschmidt, G. (2011). Plasma Oxytocin Concentration during Pregnancy is associated with Development of Postpartum Depression. *Neuropsychopharmacology, 36*(9), 1886-1893.

Skuse, D. H., & Gallagher, L. (2009). Dopaminergic-neuropeptide interactions in the social brain. *Trends in Cognitive Sciences, 13*(1), 27-35.

Sofroniew, M. V. (1983) Morphology of Vasopressin and Oxytocin Neurones and Their Central and Vascular Projections. *Vol. 60* (pp. 101-114).

Sroufe, L. A. (2005). Attachment and development: A prospective, longitudinal study from birth to adulthood. *Attachment & Human Development, 7*(4), 349 - 367.

Stein, A., Gath, D. H., Bucher, J., Bond, A., Day, A., & Cooper, P. J. (1991). The relationship between post-natal depression and mother-child interaction. *The British Journal of Psychiatry, 158*(1), 46-52. doi: 10.1192/bjp.158.1.46

Strathearn, L., Fonagy, P., Amico, J., & Montague, P. R. (2009). Adult Attachment Predicts Maternal Brain and Oxytocin Response to Infant Cues. *Neuropsychopharmacology, 34*(13), 2655-2666.

Strathearn, L., Li, J., Fonagy, P., & Montague, P. R. (2008). What's in a Smile? Maternal Brain Responses to Infant Facial Cues. *Pediatrics, 122*(1), 40-51. doi: 10.1542/peds.2007-1566

Suomi, S. J. (1997). Early determinants of behaviour: evidence from primate studies. *Br Med Bull, 53*(1), 170-184.

Swain, J. E., Lorberbaum, J. P. L., Kose, S., & Strathearn, L. (2007). Brain basis of early parent-infant interactions: psychology, physiology, and in vivo functional neuroimaging studies. *Journal of Child Psychology and Psychiatry, 48*(3-4), 262-287.

Taylor, S. E., Klein, L. C., Lewis, B. P., Gruenewald, T. L., Gurung, R. A. R., & Updegraff, J. A. (2000). Biobehavioral responses to stress in females: Tend-and-befriend, not fight-or-flight. *Psychological Review, 107*(3), 411-429. doi: 10.1037/0033-295x.107.3.411

Teti, D. M., Gelfand, D. M., Messinger, D. S., & Isabella, R. (1995). Maternal depression and the quality of early attachment: An examination of infants, preschoolers, and their mothers. *Developmental Psychology, 31*(3), 364-376. doi: 10.1037/0012-1649.31.3.364

Tost, H., Kolachana, B., Hakimi, S., Lemaitre, H., Verchinski, B. A., Mattay, V. S., . . . Meyerâ€"Lindenberg, A. (2010). A common allele in the oxytocin receptor gene (OXTR) impacts prosocial temperament and human hypothalamic-limbic structure and function. *Proceedings of the National Academy of Sciences, 107*(31), 13936-13941. doi: 10.1073/pnas.1003296107

Urban, J., Carlson, E., Egeland, B., & Sroufe, L. A. (1991). Patterns of individual adaptation across childhood. *Development and Psychopathology, 3*(4), 445-460.

Uvnäs-Moberg, K. (1998). Oxytocin may mediate the benefits of positive social interaction and emotions. *Psychoneuroendocrinology, 23*(8), 819-835.

van Londen, L., Goekoop, J. G., van Kempen, G. M. J., Frankhuijzen-Sierevogel, A. C., Wiegant, V. M., van der Velde, E. A., & De Wied, D. (1997). Plasma levels of arginine vasopressin elevated in patients with major depression. *Neuropsychopharmacology, 17*(4), 284-292. doi: 10.1016/s0893-133x(97)00054-7

Warren, S. L., Huston, L., Egeland, B., & Sroufe, L. A. (1997). Child and adolescent anxiety disorders and early attachment. *Journal of the American Academy of Child & Adolescent Psychiatry, 36*(5), 637-644. doi: 10.1097/00004583-199705000-00014

Whiffen, V. E., & Gotlib, I. H. (1993). Comparison of postpartum and nonpostpartum depression: Clinical presentation, psychiatric history, and psychosocial functioning. *Journal of Consulting and Clinical Psychology, 61*(3), 485-494. doi: 10.1037/0022-006x.61.3.485

# 4

# Postnatal Depression: When Reality Does Not Match Expectations

Carol Kauppi, Phyllis Montgomery, Arshi Shaikh and Tamara White
*Laurentian University, Sudbury, Canada*

## 1. Introduction

In popular imagery and discourse, the concept of motherhood is a mythical, magical and powerful role; however, the documented reality of many mothers' lives indicates that early parenthood does not consist solely of positive experiences (Harwood, MacLean & Durkin, 2007; Nicolson, 1999). Nevertheless, the myths of ideal mothering still prevail in contemporary society. 'Good' mothers are seen to be fulfilled in their new social role and as selflessly, happily attending to infant tasks.

This dominant ideology does not reflect the typical realities for most mothers (Barr, 2008). Indeed, for many mothers, reality involves sleepless nights, anxiety, stress, feelings of being overwhelmed and difficulties in coping. Yet women feel compelled to fit into the socially constructed mould of the good mother. Therefore, experiences that differ from the dominant perspective are often considered to stem from personal shortcomings and are perceived both by society and by women as constituting failure. Harwood et al. (2007) found that unrealistic expectations of parenthood often led to greater difficulties adjusting to the experience itself. The discrepancy between anticipated and real outcomes becomes problematic for parents in terms of their psychological adjustment and acceptance of their new reality.

The conflict between expectations and reality has been noted in the literature on motherhood and postnatal depression (Alici-Evcimen & Sudak, 2003; Beck, 2002; Mauthner, 1999; Nicolson, 1999). The incongruity between expectations of happiness and depressive symptoms—at a time that is typically regarded as joyful—further increases maternal guilt and isolation (Alici-Evcimen & Sudak, 2003; Hall & Wittkowski, 2006). Women question themselves and their worth as mothers and as individuals when their mothering experience is not what society has conditioned them to believe is acceptable. There is, therefore, a discrepancy between what is experienced and the perception of what the experience ought to be like. Hall and Wittkowski (2006) report that women perceive a need to be perfect as mothers. However, good intentions may have little impact in regard to the subjective and unpredictable realm that is motherhood.

Mauthner's (1999) research on postnatal depression found that all mothers in the study experienced some kind of conflict between their views of the mother they felt themselves to be and the mother they wanted to be. Similarly Dennis and Chung Lee (2006) found that all mothers in their study struggled to fulfill their ideal perception of motherhood while at the same time concealing their needs. They surmised that motherhood is plagued by the damaging effects of cultural norms, ideals and expectations. Consequently, mothers experiencing postnatal depression are hesitant to disclose their true feelings out of shame and perceived stigma as well as a fear of being deemed unfit for motherhood (Alici-Evcimen & Sudak, 2003; Dennis & Chung Lee, 2006).

Mauthner (1999) indicates that knowledge in regard to postnatal depression has been developed largely from within a medical model and approaches using quantitative methodologies which conceptualize postnatal depression as a disease or an illness. Research efforts have been devoted to describing, predicting, preventing and treating it. Yet Nicolson (1999) has argued that there is little empirical support indicating a biological basis for postnatal depression. McMullen and Stoppard (2006, p. 276) similarly suggest that the medical model focuses on fixing women by altering their biochemistry, personality or life circumstances; such an approach is deemed problematic:

> The consequence of such a conceptualization is that attention is not directed to what, from feminist-informed perspectives, are the sources of the problem—specifically, the structural (economic and political) conditions that affect women and how these conditions, along with gendered expectations, are brought to bear on our understandings of women's distress.

Feminist approaches seek to create theory grounded in women's experiences, language and concepts. Some authors advocate for research focused on the socially constructed, gendered values and norms that create or sustain postnatal depression (Edhborg, Friberg, Lyndh, & Widstrom, 2005; Leung, Martinson, & Arthur, 2005; Mauthner, 1999). Based on this approach, the postnatal period is similar to a period of metamorphosis for women. As women adapt to their new social roles, they also shed part of their former selves, relationships, roles and activities which are incompatible with motherhood (Van Gennep, 1960).

A common belief is that depression renders women incapable of conveying meaningful insight into their experience or of generating trustworthy accounts of their feelings (Mauthner, 1999). In contrast, within the current study, the meanings that women attribute to their experiences and daily lives can provide clearer, first hand accounts of postnatal depression and generate a more holistic understanding of subjective lived reality. The purpose of this study was twofold. The first objective was to examine women's descriptions of postnatal depression and their stated needs in order to inform the development of a peer support program. The second objective was to explore the women's perspectives on postnatal depression given their location in northern and rural contexts since much of the published postnatal literature involves women residing in large urban settings.

## 2. Method

This qualitative descriptive study is an aspect of a larger participatory action project involving women with postnatal depression, their significant others, researchers, and interdisciplinary providers. Drawing on diverse forms of knowing, the overall goal was to design a model of peer support for northern and rural women and their families experiencing postnatal depression. The subset of data used for this study was particular to women's expectations regarding motherhood, their descriptions and perceptions of postnatal depression and their needs.

### 2.1 Setting and sample

The study was conducted in four communities in northern Ontario located within a 300 kilometre radius. Within the communities, women typically only had access to primary health services. In two of the four communities, women identified a range of services such as mother-baby centres, community mental health centres and forms of peer support groups. Purposive and snowball sampling techniques were used to recruit participants. The inclusion criteria specified that the participants sought were women 18 years of age or older, French or English speaking who self-identified as having experienced postnatal depression. Verbal and written announcements about the study were distributed at various community sites such as local libraries, play centres, and posted on grocery store bulletin boards. The sample for the current chapter included 15 women.

### 2.2 Data collection

Ethical approval was obtained from the sponsoring university in northern Ontario. The topics used to guide semi-structured individual and group interviews were related to their postnatal experiences, their support needs, and barriers and solutions to peer support in postnatal depression. Each interview lasted 30 to 90 minutes and took place in a location most convenient for participants. All interviews were audio-recorded and transcribed verbatim.

### 2.3 Data analysis

Using the anonymized data sets, a thematic analysis was undertaken (Buultjens & Liamputtong, 2007; Creswell, 2007). From the transcripts of interviews, data excerpts associated with experiences of PPD and needs were identified and extracted. Feminist analysis was employed to assist in examining postnatal depression within the context of gender relations and socially constructed expectations. As Buultjens and Liamputtong (2007, p. 78) state,

> The myth of the maternal instinct can create feelings of inadequacy in mothers who do not feel overwhelming joy and love for the new child and for those who find mothering tiring and stressful. Feminist writers have challenged society's double standard where on the one hand motherhood is idealized and on the other hand it is trivialized and undervalued.

Motherhood remains a benchmark for femininity yet it is characterized by a patriarchal array of assumptions, expectations, stereotypes and impositions that dictate the dynamics of that role. Feminist analysis yields a description of social relations acknowledging gender-based oppression by identifying female experience within a social and political realm viewing women in the context of their relationships, families and communities and does not accept the status quo values and assumptions about women (Kelly, Bobo, Avery, & McLaughlin, 2004). To this end, the text was repeatedly read to code the data into categories, then group similar categories into themes. The process involves reading the verbatim transcripts, creating themes and sub-themes, aggregating the sub-themes into theme clusters and comparing the theme clusters to the original transcripts.

To address credibility, the authors regularly articulated and discussed the constructions of their perceptions of the data in an effort to check on the evolving analysis and the group decision-making processes pertaining to the identification of themes and subthemes (Creswell, 2009). Additionally, negative case analysis was employed in an effort to identify negative or disconfirming evidence.

## 3. Results and discussion

For the women in this study, the core theme was the stigma of being considered "crazy". Their struggles in the initial postnatal period were negatively influenced by fear, loss, guilt, isolation and being overwhelmed. In response to their perceived vulnerability, some sought support from within their social or professional networks. Unfortunately, this often resulted in further disengagement as they perceived being judged as "bad" or "unfit" for motherhood. Such experiences were in contrast to their expectations, as Patricia explained:

> The reason, well one of the reasons, I didn't go to my doctor and let him know is because I thought I was going nuts. And I thought that as soon as I went to my doctor and told him how I was feeling, the symptoms I was experiencing, they would take my baby away. So I had that fear that my baby was going to be taken away. I wasn't thinking rationally.

Gross (1998) proposes that Western romanticized ideologies of motherhood have an enormous impact on how women are stereotyped. Such images characterize women as sacrificing themselves for the sake of their children and husbands. Postnatal depression, defined as a personal defect and individual dysfunction, creates a 'cloak and dagger' context in which women feel the need to hide their symptoms and repress their feelings for fear of social repercussions. Mauthner (1999) found that postnatal depression occurs when women are unable to experience, express and validate their feelings and needs within supportive, accepting and non-judgmental interpersonal relationships and cultural contexts. Women feel trapped in their experience as a result of being unable to express themselves; consequently they strive to present themselves according to social and cultural expectations.

The sense that postnatal depression was something that needed to be hidden was a common experience for many of our study participants. The perception is driven by many different factors but mainly the fear of what others in society would think based on the stigma that continues to be attached to mental illness and specifically mental illness among mothers. Joanne expressed her fear of being diagnosed with postnatal depression: "I don't want to have that label because then you're associated with that behaviour." Patricia felt isolated in her experience and stated, "It would have been nice for me to know that there are other women out there feeling the same way. I am not the only, you know, crazy one. Um because at the time I did feel like I was crazy."

In the public mind, postnatal depression is associated with mental illness. Hence a diagnosis of postnatal depression stamps a woman with "craziness" which society uses to judge women as mothers and as individuals. Kristen expresses this view:

> I didn't really fit in with anything, you know. I kind of thought, well you know, [I'm] not mentally ill, but even though it is a mental illness obviously. But when you, you kinda get that stigma and that, you know, I didn't really want to fit in there I guess.

Several other participants expressed similar feelings in regard to their assumption that there would be negative public perceptions of them. Carole stated "After I found out I had it [postnatal depression] I was going to worry about what people would think of me." Patricia recalls, "People are perceiving you as, nuts, out of control, not in control of yourself, not in control of your feelings, immature. ' Like grow up, snap out of it'."

The stigma attached to the diagnosis of postnatal depression appears to dissuade women from identifying their struggle, acknowledging their needs and seeking help for their symptoms. Kristen explained this idea:

> I think it was just um, a fear of what's gonna happen you know? Like, I pretty much knew it was postpartum depression—I kinda self-diagnosed. And um, I was afraid of you know what kind of medications I might have to take and I'm breastfeeding this baby. I didn't want to take the meds. And I was getting into breastfeeding almost. There were a few of us at work that had babies all within a few months of each other. I didn't want to be the one that has postpartum depression. I was wanting to fit in with the mom and baby group thing.

Women appear to hide their feelings and experiences but often secretly hope that someone will notice and help them. Brenda stated that she was "very afraid that people could tell from the outside. Yet, I don't think they could because nobody really reached out to me." Alexandra corroborated this feeling in stating that "... nobody really asked too many questions and details about how I was really coping." Nicole explained that she attempted to manage on her own and wanted help from her husband. However, she felt guilty about asking for help and subsequently resented him for not assisting her. She states:

> He [husband] actually adds to my anxiety. Like almost 50% of my anxiety is added from him. And that's the most important support that I really want. I was doing everything but I had the supermom syndrome where [I thought] 'I can do it, I can do it.' And it took for his mom to come down and say [to him], 'What is wrong with you?' To kinda say [to him], you know, 'You gotta help here.' It took for me to have almost a total meltdown.

Riley had similar difficulties and also experienced resentment. She states, "I just felt like [I was] crazy. I was this psycho woman who wanted her house clean and her husband was just a jerk." Dobris and White-Mills (2006) reviewed a variety of implications which may stem from popular media presentations of pregnancy and childrearing. Specifically, they looked at the *What to Expect* series, a series of publications for mothers that details the expected progression of pregnancy and early childhood. These authors noted that the patriarchal positions embedded in these texts reinforce gender stereotypes of disengaged fathers who have a diminished role in the practice of childrearing. Women, therefore, are led to expect that they must sustain the role of primary caregiver to their children. Further, they argued that patriarchal positions are often so embedded in discourse that they appear invisible to the rhetorical audience. Consequently, patriarchal knowledge and assumptions continue to dictate the norms and values of motherhood.

The stigma of postnatal depression prohibits its prevalence from being known and thus sustains the myth that it is a rare and strange occurrence usually experienced by women who have some form of emotional or personal deficit. Brenda states,

> You don't hear too many stories because people like me just keep quiet. ... We need to make it more comfortable for women to talk about and to share their labour stories with anybody ... you don't really share your postpartum story with anybody.

As the data from this study show, women generally do not talk about their postnatal depression experiences and thus maintain the cloak of secrecy around a phenomenon that occurs more commonly than is perceived. Feminist analysis unveils postnatal depression as being exacerbated and sustained by a patriarchal discourse and culture that individualizes and vilifies the postnatal experiences of women. As such, women feel compelled to keep their experiences hidden. As explained in the following section, this was motivated by fear.

### 3.1 Fear

Like many women in the current study, Nicolson (1999) notes that the women in her sample did not admit to experiencing postnatal depression and referred to their experience using other terms such as feeling fed up, upset, and down. Nicolson (1999) believed that this phenomenon was indicative of women's efforts to gain personal distance from postnatal depression as a pathology discourse. The current research found that women express a variety of fears in regard to both acknowledging their experiences and seeking assistance. Once again, many women attempt to hide their struggle from the world. Kristen states that "having them know what's going on is a scary thing." For her, public knowledge of her depression created a fear that she would be perceived as a bad mother and would be forced to relinquish motherhood. Kristen stated:

> You don't want to give up that role. I am the child's mother and I think a lot of times women are afraid that if people know that they have postpartum depression, they're just going to try to step in and take over. I know that's happened to a lot of women.

Kristen's concerns are legitimate. Society has developed standards which dictate an acceptable level of parenting. Should a parent be considered sub par to that standard, child welfare agencies are mandated to intervene if the safety and well-being of a child is considered at risk. Adverse impacts of maternal depression have been found in children virtually from infancy to adolescence (Smith, 2004). Maternal mental health has been linked to child risk across cognitive, social, emotional and physical developmental areas (Cleaver, 1999; Coiro, 1998). Therefore, mothers with issues of mental health are often scrutinized in terms of their ability to provide a safe and nurturing environment for their children; there is a real possibility that children will be apprehended by child welfare services if mothers are deemed incompetent due to such issues. Women are aware of this social reality and often strive to disguise their experience for fear that their children will be removed from their care. Linda underscores the experience of fear:

> I didn't seek any community resources or anything like that so I just tried to deal with it on my own. I was afraid of saying too much and that I was going to be labelled as such and have to kind of get put through a [child welfare] system.

Thus, a primary fear of mothers in the current study was related to potential intervention by child welfare authorities. As explained above, this fear was linked to the association between postnatal depression and the stigma of mental illness. Supporting this finding, Hall and Wittkowski (2006) noted that mothers had difficulty admitting their depression and that this difficulty was further exacerbated by fears of perceived consequences that they would be admitted to a psychiatric unit or that their children would be apprehended by child welfare services. Further, Mauthner (1999) found that while women realized that motherhood was a challenging and devalued activity for which many received little support, they struggled to understand their extreme reactions and feelings of deep depression. They felt they were going mad and feared that they might one day find themselves in the local mental hospital. It appears then that women experience a fear not only of what they are feeling but also a fear in regard to the consequences that may be imposed upon them should they allow anyone to have knowledge of those feelings. The basic notion according to Mauthner (1999) is that women who suffer from postnatal depression have not been able to experience their sadness and most importantly have not been able to experience it in a context of empathetic and validating relationships. As such, many women struggle with their postnatal depression in silence and battle their symptoms in isolation.

### 3.2 Sense of loss – identity, autonomy and the physical self

A view of motherhood as a joyous and fulfilling life experience has been perpetuated over time and across various cultures. In Western societies, the planning of a pregnancy, the excitement of the revealing lines on the pregnancy test stick, the baby showers, the fuzzy stuffed animals and the ritual decorating of the baby's room in pink or blue are all behaviours designed to promote motherhood as a whimsical and beautiful time. However, the colour of motherhood is often not pretty pink or soft blue but more shades of grey and sometimes black; the latter is often experienced as a rude awakening from a glorious dream. Although most new parents realize that raising a child will pose challenges, it appears that many are not fully prepared for the scope of change that a baby will bring to their lives. Isabelle describes her experience as follows:

> So I found just the life changes, uh, were such a fundamental shift for me. And then pile on the fact that you're not sleeping either. And then pile on the fact that you're now completely responsible for a creature and it is your job to make sure that they're not totally messed up in life. That is an overwhelming responsibility.

What Isabelle describes is a feeling that her entire life has changed. It is interesting that she uses the words "pile on" several times to describe the pressures she feels to manage these new changes in her life. It appears that, for Isabelle, the stressors are cumulative and take over the life she once knew. Isabelle further states that it would have been helpful if she had been more fully aware of the realities of motherhood prior to her first hand experience so that she could have been better prepared for it. She was somewhat resentful that other mothers participate in the perpetuation of the motherhood ideal while knowing that the reality is different. She indicates that the media also play a key role in defining motherhood: "It may have been comforting to have someone say 'being a mom is not easy.' Women have been sold lies through the media about how wonderful it is your first time and second time".

Isabelle is candid and honest in expressing her shock and surprise and the feeling that she was ill informed about the experience of motherhood. Nicolson (1999) explains that women experience pleasure and pain in caring for others; the giving and receiving of love takes place alongside isolation and the resentment that they are not able (or sometimes not willing) to put themselves first. It appears that there is a sense of betrayal in terms of the social construction of motherhood in the face of its reality. Isabelle states: "I wasn't depressed. It was just that I felt like I really had the wool [pulled over my eyes]—the rug pulled from under my feet. It was based on a lie from my mother from a very young age. So I felt like I had been lied to my entire life."

The magnitude of this new role is such that women are required to immerse themselves into an alternate reality and expected to develop an altruistic existence in relation to their infant. Gross (1998) discussed the ideology of intensive mothering which promotes mothers as the ideal, preferred caretakers of children and the notion that labour intensive childrearing is best. Again, embedded within the current structure of patriarchal society, gendered roles are circumscribed and perpetuate the discourse of mother as primary caretaker and father as, at best, being in a supporting role. Nicole believes that the media contribute to the presumption that couples will take on gendered roles and promote unrealistic expectations. She states:

> One of the things I think is problematic is that there is this idea that the media puts forward—this glowing idea, golden idea, of motherhood. And then, I was waiting for it to come. And some days it still doesn't come. Like when is this supposed to arrive?

The media also perpetuate the notion that women can and should "have it all" in terms of their ability to balance motherhood with an exciting lifestyle as well as a career. Having a baby is portrayed as a milestone that will make women's lives complete. It is conceived as the epitome of fulfillment. Dobris and White-Mills (2006) found that, while some women may experience negative consequences of pregnancy and childbirth, ultimately the general consensus of mainstream society, perpetuated in part by mainstream media, is that this time in a woman's life will be perceived as perhaps the pinnacle of their lives. Parenting magazines, a source of information for many new mothers, tend to gloss over the negative, stressful and tedious aspects of motherhood and promote the wonderful joys a baby can bring to a woman's life. Although this may be the case for many, it is not always so and there are many times when the role of mother interferes with one's ability to enjoy aspects of life established prior to the birth of a baby.

For some women, a baby does not bring about a sense of completion but rather varying degrees of loss. Nicole speaks about how television mothers are portrayed in a manner that is nowhere close to the real experience. She notes that television promoted "the idea that you just wake up looking gorgeous. The baby sleeps all the time. Television does not show the screaming episode and the endless nights that you don't sleep because the child is colicky for three months. "

Our participants expressed the view that women do not often wake up looking like the attractive women portrayed in magazines. New mothers often wake up with black circles under their eyes from lack of sleep. Many women considered it to be an accomplishment to have showered and dressed at some point during the day. Media representations do not reflect who most women perceive themselves to be and subsequently they begin to become unrecognizable to themselves. An array of reality programs document a couple's journey through pregnancy, culminating in the birth and the first few days following. These programs typically denote the amazing, breathtaking experience of new life and foreshadow a world of beautiful new beginnings. They do not depict sleep deprived, tense parents and crying, sleepless babies who begin to howl when they are placed in their cribs. Olivia corroborates this realization:

> Nobody talks about bad things in regard to pregnancies. Nobody talks about it you know. It is like pregnancy and motherhood or fatherhood or parenthood is supposed to be beautiful but the reality is, it is life. It is not beautiful. It is not pretty.

The transition to parenthood and the demands of caring for a newborn infant may be destabilizing forces that elicit associated psychological effects (Horowitz, Damato, Duffy, & Solon, 2005). Adapting to the changes that a baby brings is difficult because the changes are so drastic (Nicolson, 1999). Not only are parents adjusting to their new responsibilities, new roles and new lifestyles, they are usually doing so on very little sleep. Initially at least, parents' lives revolve around their new baby. No longer are they responsible only for themselves; now they must consistently place the needs of their child or children before their own. Gruen (1990) describes the postnatal period as transitional in nature and characterized by great changes. It is a time where roles, patterns, and relationships are renegotiated. She likens this change to culture shock, where former coping mechanisms are no longer applicable and new ones have not yet been developed. The fears surrounding this unfamiliar state of self and lack of trust in the new roles can be alarming. For people who are accustomed to being in control of their time and lives, the unpredictability of new infants and their own affective states can be disconcerting.

Alici-Evcimen and Sudak (2003) describe childbirth as a decisive biological, social and psychological event with concomitant physiological, interpersonal and intrapsychic demands. When defined in this manner, one can understand the all encompassing nature of this life event. Women expect to feel that their lives are now complete and not as though life as they knew it is over. Chen, Wang, Chung, Tseng, and Chou (2006) indicate that depression in the postnatal period may be seen as a problem of adjustment to new social and personal circumstances. Women must redefine themselves in relation to their children.

Our participant, Isabelle, believes that there is a need for women to be fully informed about the realities of motherhood in an effort to increase their ability to adjust to the experience. She states, "I just think that there is a real awareness required at large about what it means to be a mom. We just have very unrealistic expectations about motherhood and what that means." In general, it appears that the social construction of motherhood which permeates contemporary society sets women up to develop a sense of failure when reality does not meet expectations. Women are socialized to anticipate the gains and positive aspects that infants will bring to their lives and this anticipation clouds any thoughts about the losses that may also ensue.

Fatima recalls her experience of being bothered with the responsibilities of motherhood. She states, "I remember just being tired of having to pack a diaper bag every time I went somewhere. I was getting really annoyed with being a mom."

Fatima resented aspects of the obligation to provide child care. The day to day activities of child care can become tedious and time consuming. Whereas previously one was generally able to make decisions and leave the home without notice or forethought, having a child requires planning, preparation and accommodation that can often be exhausting. For some, the adjustment to this new lifestyle and the imposed losses are among the most daunting tasks of motherhood. Isabelle reinforces this view:

> I have to wonder how many of my symptoms would have cropped up if I was getting eight hours of sleep at night and there was no change to my restrictions in terms of my freedom. Because, all of a sudden, you have a baby and you can't go places that you would want to go when you can go because they're sleeping again so you can't leave. So I found such a huge adjustment in my life. All of a sudden I couldn't even decide when I could go to the grocery store.

These sentiments are understandable given that first time mothers have often lived an egocentric existence prior to the birth of the child. Then, instantly, they are thrust into the position of provider and caregiver to a child—not temporarily as perhaps they had done when babysitting in the past—but on a full-time basis, 24 hours a day, seven days a week. The added reality is that this job, and their commitment to it, will prevail for at least the next 16 to 18 years. In essence, life as they knew it is over and they must now adjust to their new life. Therefore, within the context of expectation versus reality, there is also, in many cases, a sense of loss over one's autonomy and identity. A new mother must face the reality that the person she once was is gone. Mothers must now shift and mould themselves into the role of mother, in many respects abandoning their former identities.

The current data also showed that women experienced both a sense of loss in terms of social identity and independence and in terms of physical self. For many women, the physical changes to their bodies during and after childbirth are a significant source of stress. Weight gain and stretch marks are but two of the many possible physical repercussions of pregnancy. In a society focused on beauty and the feminine ideal, many women struggle with their changing bodies and altered physical appearance. Georgia had a difficult time feeling confident about her appearance because of the changes that her body had endured. She became very self-conscious about her physicality and a sense of lost beauty added to her unhappiness with motherhood. Georgia recalled being uncomfortable with her appearance and becoming self-critical. She struggled with finding things to wear stating, "Oh well, I don't look good in that because I am still dealing with a belly and everything seems to be leaking." There is social pressure to gain a set amount of weight during pregnancy which is deemed acceptable within a limited, prescribed range. Comments made to pregnant women such as "you are all belly" are meant as a compliment to the woman for gaining only the socially acceptable amount of weight. After the birth, there is an expectation that women need to work hard to regain their pre-pregnancy figure. Women strive to lose their baby weight in a race to fit into their old clothes, a goal which is not easily achieved. However, the expectation is that this is what a woman must do. Women's worth is measured in terms of their ability to fit into a socially constructed mould and this expectation adds to the pressure and stress experienced by new mothers.

Unfortunately, the power of social acceptance is strong and, at a time when women are feeling tired and vulnerable, the pressure to conform can elicit an array of negative self thoughts. Women look at themselves and they look at other women and their perceptions are registered at face value failing to take into consideration external factors and varying circumstances. As a result, women may lose their self-esteem, become self conscious and internalize feelings which perpetuate a negative experience of motherhood. Dobris and White-Mills (2006) propose that women may often compare their own lived experiences to those ideals promoted by mainstream culture and they may attempt to restructure their experiences more similarly to what they perceive to be the norm. Further they suggest that, for these women, such restructuring may reaffirm their choices and subsequent actions or create a situation of alienation as women construct themselves as "less than." Georgia describes her experience at a mother's group as serving to increase her negative self thoughts. She compared herself to the other mothers and ultimately felt inadequate. Georgia states that she observed other mothers and subsequently developed a negative self-assessment:

> Like [seeing] a perfect mom going in there with a perfect baby and being like, completely made up and happy, happy, happy and everything great. And me feeling like crap and looking at her and thinking 'Ok now I feel really, really badly.'

Melissa describes a similar experience of comparison with other mothers, stating that:

> Everyone else has it all together. You know, [I asked] 'what is wrong with me?' Those conversations tend to be in that group and they seem so in tune with their baby. On the other hand, me and my baby clash with them and you have a sense that you are not holding it together.

The struggle to maintain the self while sustaining an infant's life was common throughout much of the data. Fatima states that "It seems that I hadn't brushed my teeth for like a few days. Self-care was falling behind." New mothers often become so focused on caring for the infant that they do not take the time to care for themselves in even the most basic of ways. Additionally, within the current gendered society, fathers are not expected to take an extensive role in childrearing but are commended if they choose a supportive role. The task of childcare typically rests almost exclusively on the shoulders of women. Melissa found that her mental and physical resources were exhausted. "I was so emotionally and physically exhausted that I hit the pillow and was out. Then the next day I woke up and I was just [feeling] no energy. I was just like a zombie."

She also expressed a fear that her former self was lost forever:

> I never thought my mom would be able to go back home. She, you know lived [a far distance] away. She didn't think she'd ever be able to go home and I never thought I'd be able to work again. I just, you know, I just didn't think I was going to be myself again.

Many new mothers exist in an isolated world characterized by a routine involving feeding the baby, changing the baby, soothing the baby and attending to the baby's every perceived need. Often the needs of the mother fall by the wayside and this situation ultimately serves to increase the intensity of her struggle with the adjustment to motherhood. Nicole questioned "How do you take time for yourself? How do you get motivated to do that?"

According to Nicolson (1999), motherhood alters women's lives socially, emotionally and economically. With any change comes the need for adjustment and since the human experience is subjective in nature, one's response to change will also be subjective. Women adjust to motherhood in differing ways and within differing timeframes. Not every mother has the same constellation of circumstances and adaptive factors. Therefore, adjustment is also contingent on a variety of personal and social variables. While individual stress may not solely affect a woman's psychological well-being, the cumulative effect of multiple daily stressors potentially affects a woman's adaptability in the larger context of her environment (Page & Wilhelm, 2007).

Feminist research, and qualitative research in particular, has found that the postnatal losses of autonomy and time, along with transformations in personal and occupational identity, body image and appearance, sexuality, and relationships all figure prominently in the experience of postnatal depression (Beck, 2002; Nicolson, 1999). Nicolson (1999) theorized that social prohibitions preventing women from openly grieving the losses and changes that accompany their transition to motherhood underlie postnatal depression in Western cultures. The postnatal period can be a time during which women struggle to reconcile the past and the present.

### 3.3 Feeling overwhelmed

As stated above, often women become so focused on caring for the child that the remainder of their existence becomes pressed to the background. Their entire being revolves around the baby and begins to consume them. Yet challenges are inevitable and, as our current research shows, feelings of inadequacy perpetuated by an unattainable social standard of the motherhood ideal lead women to feel pressured to conform to established standards; this in turn leads to feelings of being overwhelmed by the scope of the responsibility. Brenda reports the following:

> I started having real anxiety over being alone with [my infant child] and feeling very overwhelmed with the care. I really just needed somebody with me all the time. It was a real anxiety panic attack kind of feeling—just huge feelings of being overwhelmed and not knowing what to do, where to go.

Similarly, Alexandra describes her experience of being overwhelmed as follows:

> At the beginning it was a lot of intrusive thoughts about my health. I would have a headache and then ask myself 'What's going on?' There must be something really wrong. Then that would just escalate. Then it would be just you know a stomach pain. Then I would just get anxious about that. So that was the first emotional thoughts I had. After that it went into just being very fatigued, being depressed and crying for nothing. I was just being really anxious; like going out was a difficulty and having people over was difficult. And just feeling I needed help or couldn't do what I needed to do for my child.

The reality is that mothers are typically the primary caregivers to their children for at least the first year after birth. Although some fathers fill a primary role and even take parental leave from their employment, this is often not the case. Generally, fathers and extended family members are expected to take on a supportive role in assisting the mother with the overall caregiving and go about their daily business with relatively little interference, disturbance or additional tasks. However, mothers at home caring for their infants often feel alone and unassisted while devoting themselves to an alternate reality. The expectation is that mothers are to go about their daily business and, at the same time, take on the all encompassing task of childcare. Georgia recalls her experience as follows: "You hear stories from way back when. Moms just did it. They had no choice. They did it all with six or seven kids on their hips. They didn't have a choice whether they felt bad or were crying."

Dennis and Chung-Lee (2006) found that the rationale for women's lack of disclosure in regard to their depression was their assumption that they were expected to cope with it. Our participant, Olivia, made a similar observation stating that:

> I had no time for anything. I remember there were moments I would walk into the bedroom and just wake him [husband] up by crying because I was so overwhelmed with the demanding physical work of taking care of my child.

Barr (2008) notes that being depressed interferes with a person's functioning ability and, therefore, the moments of happy mothering can be infrequent for mothers who have a mental health disorder. Our participant, Patricia, states:

> I remember a lot of the negative aspects in his first year of life. I feel I was cheated out of his first year of life because I was there but I wasn't there. And I did [care for the child] like I bathed [the child], I changed [the child's] diaper; [the child] never went a day without being fed. I would go out on occasions with [the child] in the winter time, although it was very difficult. But I can't remember the good things. I can't remember the good times; I can just remember me in the bathtub in a foetal position crying.

Women are pulled in all directions. They are expected to care for their new babies while maintaining all other areas of their lives. The expectation is that the role of mother is a natural transition easily incorporated into women's everyday lives. However, the reality is that motherhood often involves many new tasks which ultimately become priorities for which women must find additional time and energy to fulfill. Leung et al. (2005) found that women felt frustrated and suffered from a strong sense of failure because they considered themselves incompetent. Yet there is little sympathy or empathy for the unrealistic expectations that define motherhood. The expectation is that women just need to do it without complaint because that is what women do. The social construction of motherhood and the role of women in a gendered, patriarchal society prevail and subsequently set the stage for many women to become overwhelmed.

Throughout the data, there was an indication that the feeling of being overwhelmed was perpetuated by a sense that motherhood brings about a new and often challenging reality. Patricia states:

> After [my child] was born I started seeing commercials on the television and it talked about like you're in a maze and you're trying to climb these stairs to get out of the maze and you can see the light but you can't. Whenever you get close to it, it's not there. You have to turn again and you just can't get out. And that's exactly how I felt.

Georgia questioned whether "it was going to get better" while Melissa describes her experience as having a "sense of hopelessness." Nicole reiterates this sentiment stating that "you feel as hopeless as you can in your life." Women become so consumed by managing the many new facets of their lives that they wonder when they are going to have time to breathe again. Riley states, "You feel like you are in a hole and there is no grip. You just keep falling." Motherhood is a juggling act and women are thrown more and more balls that they must attempt to keep in the air. Isabelle expressed uncertainty in not knowing "how much of depression is heightened by the fact that everything in your life is turned upside down?" What develops for many women is the sense that they need to pick up the pieces of their lives; except now, they are unsure where many of those pieces go and this adds to their feelings of being overwhelmed with their new reality.

### 3.4 Guilt

The stigma of the bad mother, of not being good enough, and the guilt of somehow failing as an individual evolved as a significant theme within the data. Mauthner (1999) found this in her research as well stating that her participants each experienced a different set of conflicts reflecting their own notions and constructions of the "good mother." In their study of depression, McMullen and Stoppard (2006) found that women implicated gender-based expectations of what constitutes a "good woman, wife and mother" in their understandings of depression. They discussed the burden of expectations to be a 'perfect' woman, wife or mother; it was often understood that these expectations were unrealistic but women still attempted to achieve them even to the point where they could no longer do so. The characteristics of the 'good mother' varied between cultural and interpersonal contexts depending on the beliefs, values and norms that had been internalized in each participant. For some, a good mother is one who stays home and cares for her children full-time, taking them to playgroups and mother-infant yoga; for others, a good mother is one who breastfeeds her child; while for others, a good mother is one who is able to strike a balance between career and home life. The perception of a "good mother" is subjective and shaped by culture, interpersonal interactions and life experiences. Mauthner (1999) found that each mother experiences a different set of conflicts reflecting her own notion and construction of the good mother. Within the current study, Fatima describes her mothering experience as follows:

> I had a bit of shame when I was first going through it. I felt like I was failing as a mother and there was something wrong with me. And even when I had feelings that I

> wasn't bonding with [the child] I was feeling guilty for it. Cause I'm like um, 'I'm not a good mom.' I saw it as a weakness as a mom to be going through what I was going through. You know I don't feel like I'm connecting with [the child]. I don't feel that connection with [the child].

Women receive messages both verbally and non-verbally in regard to the nature of social expectations surrounding motherhood. Kraus and Redman (1986) state that, even if the family realistically anticipates the stresses of parenthood, the cultural context holds yet another layer of potential contributors to postnatal depression by defining appropriate feelings and behaviours for new mothers. Women develop an ideal notion of motherhood and subsequently place extreme expectations upon themselves in measuring their circumstances according to the socially constructed standard. Behaviours and circumstances which portray anything less than this ideal are perceived to reflect weakness and failure both as a mother and as a woman. When they experience difficulty managing, women feel as though they have failed themselves, failed their children, failed their families and failed society. Isabelle states that "there's definitely a fear of letting people down and being called a bad mother."

Women carry guilt in relation to their perception that they are not good enough. Mauthner (1999) describes her understanding that mothers seem caught between two opposing voices. One set of voices reflects mothers' expectations of themselves and their interpretations of cultural norms and values surrounding motherhood while another set of voices seems to be informed by the mothers' actual, concrete, everyday experiences of mothering their particular children and in the particular circumstances in which they find themselves. When they experience depression, mothers find it difficult to accept these grounded feelings and experiences. Because the latter conflict with their expectations, they feel they must be doing something wrong and they try to change themselves in order to live up to the ideals of the good mother. Patricia explains that she had expectations which she placed upon herself but that were essentially imposed by her perception of society's expectations. She further states, "I was going through a lot of emotional challenges. I was crying a lot. I was basically just taking care of my child's basic needs and that was it. I found myself wanting to sleep a lot [and] just feeling like I was a rotten mother."

Additionally, there is guilt in regard to what women perceive they should feel and the actuality of what they are experiencing. Linda states that "I believed I must be a terrible mother to be having these feelings. 'Why am I not so happy about it [motherhood]?' Gruen (1990) proposes that depression in response to death, divorce, or job loss is culturally acceptable, whereas depression in response to the arrival of a child is not culturally approved. The social stigma and resulting shame, embarrassment, and fear prevent families from seeking help when they experience symptoms of depression. The guilt then surfaces when women do not feel the way they expected to feel and when they do not feel the way that society expects them to feel. Buultjens and Liamputtong (2007) found that Western culture stipulates that women are to have babies, that they should want to have babies and that mothering is happy experience. If a woman disrupts this assumption by being unhappy and depressed, she challenges the fundamental societal understanding of femininity and maternity. Such understandings affirm a patriarchal vantage point for assessing both the "good" and the "bad" mother, according to Dobris and White-Mills (2006).

Our participant Olivia finds it finds it difficult to reconcile her feelings and experiences with her reality and recalls that, "it didn't make sense to be with this healthy, beautiful child. And he did nothing wrong. 'What's going on with me? Why does this not make me happy? Why is it unfulfilling?' Hall and Wittkowski (2006) found that women often felt unjustified in their depression which was confusing for them and often led to increased feelings of guilt and low mood. Kraus and Redman (1986) found that some of the common cultural myths about motherhood contend that it is a woman's ultimate fulfillment associated with an indescribable joyfulness, that a woman will immediately feel love for her baby and that a woman will intuitively know how to parent. Yet, women appear to feel as though they are being judged when they do not share these experiences.

Our participants feel as though they are under scrutiny and are measured against an unattainable standard of perfection. Riley states, "you feel like everyone is looking at you. You're crying over something. 'Oh my God she's crying again.' We're so hard on ourselves too [expecting] to be the perfect mom." Helen discussed her postnatal depression experience and advised that, her perception was that "you're not supposed to have these problems. Good mothers don't have these problems." She describes postnatal depression as a vicious cycle and believes that feelings of guilt experienced by women when they perceive that they do not meet the ideal mother standard lead directly to feelings of depression. She states:

> The guilt actually makes you do stuff that you wouldn't [otherwise do]… you get more upset because you're upset and then the ball gets rolling. [I believed that] the guilt somehow caused it [postnatal depression]. If I was better at this or that or the other thing I wouldn't have this problem.

Patricia individualized her experiences as well and internalized the negative connotations of her feelings. She states that:

> I felt that like I was inadequate as a wife and mother. I felt like I was weak because everyone I knew that had babies never had any problems. They had a good pregnancy, they had nice babies. They were healthy, they went back to work and everything was fine.

A woman's worth is measured against a socially constructed ideal based in patriarchal ideology that defines women's existence. Unfortunately, this ideal is institutionalized within society promoting a social climate where the expectations placed on mothers create a skewed reality. When reality does not meet the expectation, guilt is internalized and breeds a variety of negative self thoughts which in turn can create or increase feelings of depression. Helen states: "I believe a positive sense of self is from within. No matter how often everyone is telling you, 'You're a good mom' it is irrelevant if you don't think you are."

These findings support those of Mauthner (1999) who found that, during their depression, women found it difficult to let go of their images and ideals of motherhood and criticized themselves on moral grounds. There was a pervasive sense of what they should be feeling, what they ought to be experiencing versus what they actually felt were, respectively, the right and wrong ways to mother.

Some researchers have found that maternal self-efficacy protects against the development of postnatal symptomology (Coleman & Karraker, 1997; Seguin, Potvin, St. Denis, & Loiselle, 1999). Research conducted from a feminist perspective has related postnatal depression to the challenges women face in achieving a sense of maternal competency or realizing idealized expectations of motherhood (Beck, 2002). Rubin's (1984) seminal qualitative study of pregnant and postnatal women described how the gap between the realities of motherhood and women's idealized expectations of maternity result in self deprecation and depression. Subsequently, a woman's sense of competence as a parent, satisfaction with parenting, her focus on the infant and the amount of experienced life change will either strengthen or weaken her feelings of self-efficacy during the postnatal adaptation (Horowitz et al., 2005). Patricia corroborates these sentiments and states:

> I told my husband that I was going to leave him. I said, 'I am not a good enough wife. I am not a good enough mother.' I was literally going to go to the bank to get enough money for bus ticket and just take a bus anywhere. And I didn't know what I would do when I got wherever I was going. I just wanted to get out of their life cause I thought he would be better off marrying someone else and someone else would be a better mother and a better wife.

In addition to guilt in a general sense which was experienced by many of the women in the current study, guilt was also described in more specific expectations of mothering. Breastfeeding appeared to be an area in which a number of women experienced a variety of negative and stressful emotions. The medical community actively promotes breastfeeding with slogans such as "Breast is best" and community agencies such as La Leche League are organized to assist women and their babies in ensuring that successful breastfeeding is sustained. Breastfeeding is a behaviour that is considered preferable within the scope of good mothering. However, as some of our participants stated, women may choose not to breastfeed or decide to do so but struggle with the process. Alexandra indicated that breastfeeding was challenging. It appears that, for her, breastfeeding was yet another stressor in her new motherhood experience and an opportunity for her to feel guilt because she was struggling. Helen states, "It seems like the rule of thumb is to really stick to it [breastfeeding] for four months or six months. At six months it's like, 'That's it, you are done. You are done. You did good job." This is another area in which women feel compelled to place expectations upon themselves and to comply with social values that may not be conducive to their own emotional well-being; yet these expectations are perceived by them to be essential to their ability to conform. Women may not breastfeed their babies because they want to do so but proceed with it because of social pressures. Patricia states:

> I have nothing wrong with breastfeeding you know. All the more power to you if you breastfeed. I choose not to, not because I can't [but] because I don't feel comfortable with it. And they basically, in a nut shell, they said everything but you're a rotten mother because you choose not to breastfeed. They have a La Leche League and it's a group to support women that breastfeed. I feel like there should be a group supporting parents that decide to give formula to their kids. I feel like going up on a stage and screaming, 'You know what? I am still a good mother even though I decide to give formula to my child.' I found this played a role too in how I perceived myself as being a mother. I felt like the society shunned me because I was feeding my baby formula. I was going through depression. I was just a rotten person all in all.

Nicole also expressed the view she felt pressure to breastfeed and that this added a negative dimension to her experience. She states:

> I saw this little drop of colostrum so I'd pump, pump, pump, pump, pump and then still pumping when I got home. I pumped whenever I felt full. In the back of my head I felt guilty because I thought I might have to bottle feed. And I felt this, and that added a lot of stress. I knew the benefits of breastfeeding but what if you can't do it. Don't stress about it.

Breastfeeding was equated with coming closer to that ideal mother. Instead of breastfeeding being a comfortable choice, it appeared that some women felt pressured to breastfeed despite the fact that the practice added to their stress. They felt an obligation based on the socially dictated theory that a good mother breastfeeds.

Women also felt guilt in regard to the impact that their postnatal depression had on both their immediate and extended family. They felt as though they were failing their families and burdening them with their personal difficulties. Helen felt guilt in regard to her husband and states:

> My husband is at a loss. This is not what he expected either. We were both kind of um trying to deal with it. He is trying to deal with me as well as the baby and everything. I'm trying to deal with me, the baby and him. He is trying to deal with the rest of the world and his job and all these other things that ah he has a life too.

Ellen also spoke about a similar experience and states:

> I felt a lot of guilt toward my husband. This made it hard for me to just let go of the bad feelings and just let myself feel bad until I could start to feel better. [I would have benefitted from] a lot of physical support—relieve my husband so that I wouldn't feel so guilty.

Many of our participants acknowledge that postnatal depression has far reaching effects on the majority of their social relationships. Georgia felt guilt about how her experience would impact on her own mother and states "I was nervous about letting her know [mother] because then I knew she'd be more worried about me." Although spouses and extended family can be strong sources of support for women experiencing postnatal depression, the data indicates that they can also directly or indirectly add to the guilt and stress experienced by women.

Postnatal depression can be adequately managed and women can experience reduced symptoms through the use of anti-depressant medication. However, the data in the current study indicate that many women are opposed to taking medication to address their needs for a variety of reasons. Fatima states that she "saw it as a sign of weakness to go for help or to go on medication". She had difficulty acknowledging that her experience was beyond her control and that recovery would require assistance. For others, such as Isabelle, the idea of proceeding to take medication and accept intervention was equated with a sense that she would lose control of her affect. Isabelle stated that "maybe I think I'm all powerful but I don't want to have to go the medication route." She worried about the loss of self-control:

> Part of it is you want to control your own life, your own world. As soon as you introduce drugs into this, you question, 'Will it change me?' 'How will it change me?'

> 'Am I going to be the same person?' 'Am I going to become a drone?' 'What's going to happen to my highs and lows?' Maybe I don't really want to lose my highs.

Most people prefer not to rely on pharmaceutical assistance for their day to day functioning. There is also stigma attached to the need for anti-depressive medication. Thus not only is there stigma in regard to the condition of postnatal depression, there is stigma in regard to one of its effective interventions. As such, many women are opposed to addressing their experience through medication. Melissa states that: "As soon as he said medication I was just like "Whoo!" Up went the wall." She did not want to discuss the matter as the stigma of medical intervention precluded her ability to consider its benefits.

### 3.5 Isolation and the need for support

One of the most evident experiences disclosed by study participants was the positive impact of access to support in increasing their ability to manage while struggling with postnatal depression. Women spoke about various forms of formal and informal supports both within group settings and in one-on-one interactions. It appears that support was highly valued and beneficial in assisting women both in concrete ways and on an emotional level. Seagrist (2008) found that there is substantial evidence that participating in a support group has a positive effect on well-being. The group can serve as a resource for overcoming isolation and expanding informal support networks. It also may provide a sense of hope to counterbalance situational depression arising from losses and other traumatic experiences and encourages sharing feelings of intense emotional reactions as well as new ways of coping with problematic life events. Paris and Dubus (2005) found that new mothers experienced isolation and loneliness that often led to disconnection. Our participant, Patricia, stated that: "I felt so isolated and thought I was the only one going through this." Because mothering often occurs within the walls of the home, women sometimes feel alone and separated from the rest of the world. For women experiencing postnatal depression the current data indicate that support groups allowed women to feel less isolated in their struggle and allowed them to develop an openness to revealing their experience. Involvement alleviated some of the stigma associated with postnatal depression and facilitated discussion in regard to managing. Donna had not yet participated in a support group but expressed an opinion about this:

> Support would be a place that you can go where people understand what's going on and um telling you that you're not crazy…[It would also be a place that would] give you coping strategies… the biggest thing though is just knowing that you're not crazy and that there are other people that are like you that are going through [it]. The biggest thing would be other women who understand.

This sense of relief experienced by women in terms of their newfound ability to talk about how they were feeling and to obtain some validation of their feelings within an environment of acceptance was both enticing and beneficial for many of the study participants. Alexandra felt support groups helped her:

> The best thing for me was just to open up about it as I was feeling anxious a lot. I always found that after I talked to someone, anybody, I just felt less anxious. I felt better about it. It was actually a good way to help other moms open up and say 'Yeah, you know what, I can relate or I think I went through the same thing.'

Brenda also experienced the benefit of support groups and stated that it was comforting to her: "Other people had pretty similar stories and that was a big help because it still feels like a lot of stigma with mental illness. I wanted to deal with my depression within a group of like-minded people".

Support groups then appear to remove some of the sense of stigma of postnatal depression and reduce feelings of isolation. As well it allows the opportunity for women to share their stories of coping. Participation allows them to work through various strategies and provides a sense of hope where perhaps there had been little or none. Carole states that support groups were beneficial for her: "Just hearing that someone else has gone through it and hearing other people's stories. You come to realize that you are not as bad off or as alone as you thought".

Ellen also expresses this sentiment: "I guess that I'm not alone. Just to hear other people's coping skills is helpful." In a sense, support groups are often effective because they can normalize emotions and experiences by exploring commonalities. By normalizing postnatal depression, those related experiences that women described as guilt, fear or shame are minimized. Joanne stated that attending support groups "made it more manageable, almost more normal for you. You didn't feel like you were going crazy." Helen indicated that support groups helped her realize that: "… you're not the only one. … There really are people out there and they do have the same problems that I have. They're really functioning and some of them are functioning better".

What Helen found within the group was a glimmer of hope that she was going to survive her postnatal experience. This realization had an impact on Melissa as well, as she recalled that "you know from the mothers who were kind of in recovery, they've gotten over it. You get a sense that it does get better."

For some women, involvement in a support group assisted them in addressing the experience within their families. Helen enjoyed speaking to the women in the support groups because she could see "that some of them have the same symptoms as you do and some of them have different ones. There is no right answer or wrong answer." She further stated that the support group allowed her to realize that postnatal depression can remain "a family secret if you want it to be but, if you don't want it to be, it doesn't have to be anymore." For some, support groups offer hope and provide optimism. Kristen states that the groups: "just kinda normalize it for the family. If it normalizes everything and maybe you wouldn't feel so weird talking about it with your family—maybe".

Linda concurs stating that, "you see a normal woman with a normal family, a job, and everything. It is just something that happens sometimes." Abrams and Curran (2007) found postnatal depression is negatively correlated with social support thus supporting the theory that postnatal depression is related, to a large extent, to psychosocial and environmental stressors. However, because of the on-going stigma, misinformation and secrecy that envelopes postnatal depression, women often struggle alone; loneliness can sustain itself and become a dark place where women cannot find their way out. Support groups afford the possibility of shedding some light on the experience, opening the door to communication and offering a path to recovery.

## 4. Conclusion

The Diagnostic and Statistical Manual of Mental Disorders (DSM-IV-TR) of the American Psychiatric Association does not describe postnatal depression as a category but it is listed under the broad spectrum of general depression. Yet postnatal depression, viewed as a separate condition, often remains undiagnosed and untreated (Dennis & Chung Lee, 2006). "Risk factors for postnatal depression that are commonly reported in the literature include maternal characteristics such as being single, younger, of low socio-economic status, being anxious, having a history of depression and exposure to recent life stress" (Howell, Mora, & Leventhal, 2006, pp. 149). These variables are static factors. They are, for the most part, unchangeable in the short term. However, when we look beyond an individualistic understanding of women's experiences and specifically of postnatal depression, we discover an array of situational factors. Nicolson (1999) states that clinical practice and popular knowledge in this regard appear to be based on belief, myth and a body of contentious empirical evidence; however, the nature and definition of postnatal depression remains largely unknown. Nicolson (1999) proposes that perhaps postpartum depression is a normal response to the fundamental changes a woman experiences as a result of pregnancy, childbirth and mothering. Abrams and Curran (2007, p. 292) make a similar argument:

> Feminists have argued that the medical model tends to pathologize women's negative postpartum affective experiences instead of recognizing that these experiences are normative and potentially inevitable. They have maintained that the physical trauma of and recovery from childbirth, sleep deprivation, new responsibilities, and the need to quickly master new skill sets would produce emotional disturbances in anyone.

When viewed through the lens of feminist standpoint theory, it is plausible that the current social and cultural climate serves to thrust upon women unattainable expectations while promoting a skewed reality in regard to the experience of motherhood. It generally sets women up to fail and then condemns them for their apparent failures. However, Mauthner (1999) argues that consideration of postnatal depression as a normal response to motherhood trivializes and minimizes feelings which mothers themselves experience as terrifying and abnormal.

In light of the current findings, it appears that, on some level, both theories are relevant. It is not surprising that many women experience postnatal depression given the context of their experiences. However, in terms of normalization, it appears that it is not the condition of postnatal depression that is normalized but the structure of society that perpetuates its existence. There is currently an acceptance of the status quo which allows women's lives to be defined by values and norms which are not their own but those created by dominant discourse that fails to acknowledge the realities of women's experiences. Buultjens and Liamputtong (2007) state that the overall recognition of depression is an indication of change in societal acceptance of a mother's inability to cope automatically with the life-altering transition associated with motherhood. However, the myth of blissful parenthood is still embedded in a large proportion of our society, stigmatizing anxiety and depression after childbirth.

The findings of our study are similar to those of Abrams and Curran (2007) in terms of the notion that nearly all mothers experiencing postnatal depression symptoms hesitated to disclose their feelings to others due to fear that they will be judged, labelled as "crazy" or rejected by family and friends. Abrams and Curran (2007) also state that shame and guilt associated with the failure to fulfill idealized maternal expectations make mothers less inclined to seek help for postnatal depression. Additionally, the current study is consistent with prior research conducted by Haslam, Pakenham and Smith (2006) who found that social support and maternal self-efficacy are inversely related to postnatal depression and appear to protect against the development of postnatal symptomology. Our findings also corroborate the notion put forward by Howell et al. (2006) that the negative impact of the functional limitations of postnatal depression on mothers' emotional states can be reduced by a supportive social environment and self confidence in carrying out daily activities. Overall, the findings of the current study indicate that women's experiences of postnatal depression extend beyond a medical model of individual pathology and are best understood in relation to the social and cultural climate in which they occur.

## 5. Implications for practice

When expectations lie in contrast to reality, not only are women's realities often surreal, the characterization of the experiences associated with postnatal depression can be identified as significant barriers to both diagnosis and treatment. It can be assumed that the prevalence of postnatal depression is not truly known as many women do not acknowledge or report their experiences in relation to the perceived social repercussions of their disclosures. In terms of adequately assessing and subsequently serving women with postnatal depression, health care professionals and community service providers must obtain a holistic understanding of women's lives looking beyond a medical model towards a thorough awareness of those social and cultural influences that constitute a woman's lived reality.

When we observe, within the findings of the current study, the experiences of loss, guilt, shame, stigma, fear and inadequacy with which many women struggle postpartum, it is evident that the impact of such experiences can be debilitating and often paralyzing for women and have far reaching effects on their personal and social functioning. When reality does not match expectations and the expectations are not realistic, women struggle to redefine their reality but must do so under social and cultural pressures which serve to destabilize them. The instability can result in an internal battle with the self and the context of one's life. There is a need to foster awareness in regard to the experience of new mothers, the pressures placed upon women entering motherhood and the social and personal expectations which create and sustain a reality that contributes to impairments in individual and family functioning. Society in general needs to be educated about the nature of postnatal depression in order for the related stigma to be removed, thus allowing women's struggles to become less isolated. In removing the cloak of secrecy and shame around the experience of postnatal depression, the opportunity may arise for women's realities to be unveiled and their needs addressed in a manner that is timely, appropriate and beneficial to the overall health and well-being of women and families.

Lastly, the current findings evidenced the benefit of support programs for women experiencing postnatal depression. Overwhelmingly, women expressed their view that their postpartum symptomology—such as feelings of isolation and guilt and fears that they were going crazy—were reduced through their ability to share their experiences with individuals who were understanding and to whom they could relate. The availability of postnatal support groups may be an effective community intervention which can have a positive impact on the ability of mothers to express their feelings and develop coping strategies that can assist them in navigating their way out of their depression. Unfortunately, access to postnatal support groups is not universal. For many women residing in rural, remote or northern communities, the reality is that such services simply do not exist. In light of the current findings, the benefit of postnatal support groups must be highlighted and promoted in an effort to obtain resources and develop initiatives which may allow these quality services to be available to all women despite geographical location.

In viewing postnatal depression through from a feminist standpoint, it is logical that interventions should be based on feminist principles supporting women within the context of their lives through strengths-based interactions and strategies designed to empower women in all regards. Ultimately, the research findings have contributed to knowledge in regard to understanding their perceptions and providing information to guide meaningful direct service to women and families. Only when postnatal depression is understood holistically can positive change be effected for those struggling in the shadow of this phenomenon.

## 6. Implications for future research

It is noted that postnatal depression is often assessed using the Beck's Depression Inventory (BDI) and/or the Edinburgh Postnatal Depression Scale (EPDS). These are self-report scales in which women's responses determine a diagnosis. Should women choose not to disclose their struggles out of fear, shame or guilt, they may not be forthcoming in their responses to the administration of these instruments; consequently, the reality of postnatal depression is dismissed. Additionally, it is noted that the majority of the themes found in current qualitative research related to postnatal depression are not reflected in or quantified within the EPDS or BDI. It is notable that, within these standardized scales, there is no reference to feeling overwhelmed, tearful, isolated or experiencing loss. Therefore, it is proposed that those tools do not adequately measure the breadth of postnatal depression. Beck (1992) indicates that "even though a woman does not need to exhibit every symptom of postnatal depression to be diagnosed as experiencing the disorder, quantitative instruments should include the gamut of possible behavioural manifestations from which a mother can rate her symptomology" (pg. 170). Qualitative studies such as the current one can be used as a starting point for methodological research focused on developing a qualitative instrument to assess postnatal depression. In an effort to improve future methodology on the topic of postnatal depression, the development and promotion of qualitative research in this area of study is considered essential so as to provide a holistic understanding of the subjective experience of this social phenomenon.

## 7. Strengths of the study

The findings of the current study based on a sample of women in Northern Ontario are strengthened by the similarity to those found in prior research in terms of the experience of postnatal depression. Specifically, the findings were consistent with past research which found the experience of postnatal depression to be characterized by feelings of loss, guilt, shame and inadequacy. The qualitative nature of the study lends to the authenticity of the findings in that the experiences are defined by women in their own words.

## 8. References

Abrams, L. S., & Curran, L. (2007). Not just a middle class affliction: Crafting a social work research agenda on postpartum depression. *Health and Social Work, 32*(4), pp. 289-296.

Alici-Evcimen, Y., & Sudak, D. (2003). Postpartum depression. *Primary Care Update Ob/Gyn, 10* (5), 210-216.

American Psychiatric Association. (2000). *Diagnostic and statistical manual of mental disorders* (4th ed., text rev.). Washington, DC: Author.

Barr, J.A. (2008). Postpartum depression, delayed maternal adaptation and mechanical infant caring: A phenomenological hermeneutic study. *International Journal of Nursing Studies, 45* (3), pp. 362-369.

Beck, C. T. (1992). The lived experience of postpartum depression: A phenomenological study. *Nursing Research, 41* (3), 166-170.

Beck, C. T. (2002). Postpartum depression: A metasynthesis. *Qualitative Health Research, 12*(4), 453-472.

Buultjens, M., & Liamputtong, P. (2007). When giving life starts to take the life out of you: Women's experiences of depression after childbirth. *Midwifery, 23* (1), pp. 77-91.

Chen, C., Wang, S., Chung, U., Tseng, Y., & Chou, F. (2006). Being Reborn: the recovery process of postpartum depression in Taiwanese women. *Journal of Advanced Nursing, 54* (4), pp. 450-456.

Cleaver, H. (1999). *Children's needs – parenting Capacity: The Impact of Parental Mental Illness, Problem Alcohol and Drug Use and Domestic Violence on Children's Development.* London, UK: The Stationary Office.

Coiro, M.J. (1998). *Maternal depressive symptoms as a risk factor for child development in poverty.* Dissertation Abstracts International Section B: The Sciences and Engineering, 58, 7b.

Coleman, P. K., & Karraker, K. H. (1997). Self-efficacy and parenting quality: Findings and future applications. *Developmental Review, 18*, 47-85.

Creswell, J. (2007). *Qualitative Inquiry and Research Design: Choosing Among Five Traditions.* Thousand Oakes, California, USA: Sage Publications.

Creswell, J. (2009). Research *Design: Qualitative, quantitative and mixed methods approaches.* (3rd Edition).Thousand Oakes, California, USA: Sage Publications.

Dennis, C. L., & Chung-Lee, L. (2006). Postpartum depression help-seeking barriers and maternal treatment preferences: A qualitative systemic review. *Birth, 33*(4), pp. 323-331.

Dobris, C.A., & White-Mills, K. (2006). Rhetorical visions of motherhood: A feminist analysis of the What to Expect series. *Women & Language, 29*(1), pp. 26-36.

Edhborg, M., Friberg, M., Lyndh, W., & Widstrom, A.M. (2005). Struggling with life: Narratives from women with signs of postpartum depression. *Scandinavian Journal of Public Health, 33*, pp. 261-267

Gross, E. (1998). Motherhood in feminist theory. *Afflia Journal of Women and Social Work, 3*(3), pp. 269.

Gruen, D.S. (1990). Postpartum depression: A debilitating yet often unassessed problem. *Health and Social Work, 15*(4), pp. 261-270.

Hall, P., & Wittkowski, A. (2006). An exploration of negative thoughts as a normal phenomenon after childbirth. *Journal of Midwifery & Women's Health, 51*(5), pp. 321-330.

Haslam, D. M., Pakenham, K. I., & Smith, A. (2006). Social support and postpartum depressive symptomatology: The mediating role of maternal self-efficacy. *Infant Mental Health Journal, 27* (3), 276-291.

Harwood, K., McLean, N., & Durkin, K. (2007). First-time mothers expectations of parenthood: What happens when optimistic expectations are not matched by later experiences? *Developmental Psychology, 43*(1), pp. 1-12.

Horowitz, J.A., Damato, E.G., Duffy, M.E., & Solon, L. (2005). The relationship of maternal depression, attributes, resources and perceptions of postpartum experiences to depression. *Research in Nursing & Health, 28*, pp. 159-171.

Howell, E.A., Mora, P., & Leventhal, H. (2006). Correlates of early postpartum depressive symptoms. *Maternal and Child Health Journal, 10* (2), pp.149-157.

Kelly, P.J., Bobo, T., Avery, S., & McLaughlin, K. (2004). Feminist perspectives and practice with young women. *Issues in Comprehensive Pediatric Nursing, 27* (2), pp. 121-133.

Kraus, M. S., & Redman, E.S. (1986). Postpartum depression: An interactional view. *Journal of Marital and Family Therapy, 12* (1). pp. 63-74.

Leung, S. S. K., Martinson, I. M., & Arthur, D. (2005). Postpartum depression and related psychological variables in Hong Kong Chinese women: Findings from a prospective study. *Research in Nursing & Health, 28* (1), 27-38.

Mauthner, N. (1999). Feeling low and feeling really bad about feeling low: Women's experiences of motherhood and postpartum depression. *Canadian Psychology, 40* (2), pp.143-161.

McMullen, L. M., & Stoppard, J. M. (2006). Women and depression: A case study of the influence of feminism in Canadian psychology. *Feminism Psychology, 16* (3), pp. 273-288.

Nicolson, P. (1999). Loss, happiness and postpartum depression: The ultimate paradox. *Canadian Psychology, 40* (2), pp. 162-178.

Page, M., & Wilhelm, M.S. (2007). Postpartum daily stress, relationship quality and depressive symptoms. Contemporary *Family Therapy, 29*, pp. 237-251.

Paris, R., & Dubus, N. (2005). Staying connected while nurturing an infant: A challenge of new motherhood. *Family Relations, 54*, pp. 72-83.

Rubin, R. (1984). *Maternal identity and the maternal experience.* New York, USA: Springer.

Seguin, L., Potvin, L., St-Denis, M., & Loiselle, J. (1999). Socio-environmental factors and postnatal depressive symptomatology: A longitudinal study. *Women & Health, 29*, 57-71.

Seagrist, K.A. (2008). Impact of support groups on the well-being of older women. *Journal of Gerentological Social Work, 51*(2), pp. 42-52.

Smith, M. (2004). Parental mental health: Disruptions to parenting and outcome for children. *Child & Family Social Work, 9* (1), 3-11.

Van Gennep, A. (1960). *The rites of passage*. London, UK: Routledge& Kegan Paul.

# 5

# Employment During Pregnancy Protects Against Postpartum Depression

Elisabet Vilella* et al.
*Hospital Psiquiàtric Universitari Institut Pere Mata, IISPV, Universitat Rovira i Virgili, Reus, Spain*

## 1. Introduction

Postpartum depression (PPD), a disorder that has severe consequences for mother and child (Pearlstein, Howard, Salisbury, & Zlotnick, 2009), is the most common psychiatric disorder experienced by women after childbirth (McGarry, Kim, Sheng, Egger, & Baksh, 2009), with a prevalence of ~7% during the first three postpartum months (O'Hara, 2009). While different biological (Albacar et al., 2011; Brummelte & Galea, 2010; Leung & Kaplan, 2009) and genetic (Costas et al., 2010; Mahon et al., 2009; Sanjuan et al., 2008; Treloar, Martin, Bucholz, Madden, & Heath, 1999) factors have been associated with PPD, most researchers have identified a history of affective disorder, depressive episodes and anxiety during pregnancy as the principal risk factors for PPD (O'Hara, 2009; Oppo et al., 2009). Social and psychological factors such as marital discord, low social support, stressful life events and lack of marital support have been strongly associated with PPD in several studies (Beck, 2001; Chen, 2001; O'Hara, 2009), and unemployment, which has been associated with depression in the general population (Stankunas, Kalediene, Starkuviene, & Kapustinskiene, 2006), has been specifically associated with PPD (Chen, 2001; Inandi et al., 2002; Jardri et al., 2006; Lane et al., 1997; Miyake, Tanaka, Sasaki, & Hirota, 2011; Posmontier, 2008; Rubertsson, Wickberg, Gustavsson, & Radestad, 2005; Warner, Appleby, Whitton, & Faragher, 1996). However, the results of studies on the impacts of other social variables such as income (Miyake et al., 2011) and the mother's level of education (Beck, 2001; Josefsson et al., 2002; Kozinszky et al., 2011; Miyake et al., 2011) are controversial. A recent study in Japan found that full-time employment and professional or technical employment significantly reduced the risk of PPD, leading researchers to claim that it is likely that a

* Glòria Albacar[1], Rocío Martín-Santos[2,3], Lluïsa García-Esteve[3], Roser Guillamat[4], Julio Sanjuan[5], Francesca Cañellas[6], Isolde Gornemann[7], Yolanda de Diego[8], Ana Gaviria[1] and Alfonso Gutiérrez-Zotes[1]
[1]*Hospital Psiquiàtric Universitari Institut Pere Mata, IISPV, Universitat Rovira i Virgili, Reus, Spain*
[2]*Neuropsychopharmacology Program, IMIM-Parc de Salut, Barcelona, Spain*
[3]*Department of Psychiatry, Institute of Neuroscience, Hospital Clínic, IDIBAPS, CIBERSAM, Barcelona, Spain*
[4]*Coorporació Sanitària Parc Taulí, Sabadell, Spain*
[5]*Faculty of Medicine, CIBERSAM, Universitat de Valencia, Valencia, Spain*
[6]*Hospital Universitari Son Dureta, UNICS, Palma de Mallorca, Spain*
[7]*Fundación para la e-Salud, Málaga, Spain*
[8]*Hospital Carlos Haya, Málaga, Spain*

higher degree of job satisfaction protects one from PPD (Miyake et al., 2011). Furthermore, unemployment, and the attendant lack of income, during the postpartum period has been associated with lower levels of self-esteem and negative self-perception, both of which are risk factors for PPD (Chen, 2001). Absences due to sickness are more frequent in pregnant women than in non-pregnant women (A. Sydsjo, Sydsjo, & Alexanderson, 2001), and sick leave is a strong risk factor for the presence of postpartum depressive symptoms (Josefsson et al., 2002).

Neuroticism a fundamental personality trait which has also been implicated in postpartum depression (Beck, 2001), correlates with a negative perception of one's social and economic statuses and tends to intensify feelings and beliefs about illness (Alfonsi, Conway, & Pushkar, 2011). To our knowledge, no studies have assessed the relationship among employment, sick leave, personality traits and PPD. In a previous study on biological markers for PPD, we identified an association between employment, neuroticism and PPD (Albacar et al., 2011). We hypothesized that women with higher scores for neuroticism would be more frequently unemployed or on sick leave during pregnancy and, therefore, be more at risk for PPD. Conversely, we hypothesized that women who are more active during pregnancy would be less susceptible to PPD.

## 2. Materials and methods

### 2.1 Study population

Our study population was obtained from a larger multicenter prospective study of 1,804 women recruited in Spain between December 2003 and October 2004 to study genetic and environmental factors associated with PPD (Sanjuan et al., 2008). All participants volunteered, were of Spanish origin (Caucasian), were over 18 years of age and had a singleton baby. Participants with depression or other psychiatric illnesses during pregnancy were excluded from the study. Other exclusion criteria included cognitive impairments, the presence of a medical illness that prevented participation and the lack of data for any of the considered variables. Overall, 1,724 women were included in the study. The ethics committees at each of the participating hospitals approved the study.

### 2.2 Procedures

Participants were contacted 48 h postpartum at the hospital obstetric unit and invited to participate by the research team, which was comprised of clinical psychologists and psychiatrists. Upon acceptance, participants completed semi-structured interviews for the collection of socio-demographic data. Obstetric data were collected from obstetric medical records.

Socio-demographic variables included age (years), marital status (grouped as with or without partner), educational level (grouped as primary school equivalent to 9 years of education, secondary school equivalent to 13 years of education or college degree equivalent to 20 years of education), occupational status before and during pregnancy (grouped as active, e.g., employed, housewife and student, or inactive, e.g., unemployed and sick leave), type of coexistence (grouped as parents, own family or other) and perceived household income (grouped as adequate, low or very low).

Obstetric variables of interest included the presence of a medical illness, defined as the presence of any medical condition that involved either hospitalization or pharmacological treatment during pregnancy or the peripartum period. This variable was dichotomized as presence or absence.

Depressive symptoms were screened 8 weeks and 32 weeks postpartum using the validated Spanish language version of the Edinburgh Postnatal Depression Scale (EPDS) (Garcia-Esteve, Ascaso, Ojuel, & Navarro, 2003). Participants were screened at 8 weeks to accommodate mothers scheduled for a postpartum obstetric visit at this time, and most bibliographic references, including the Diagnostic and Statistical Manual of Mental Disorders IV (DSM IV), state that postpartum depression usually develops during the first 4 weeks postpartum. Depression was assessed at 32 weeks on the basis of data stating that postpartum depression can develop up to 12 months postpartum (O'Hara, 2009). A baseline assessment was conducted 48 h postpartum when the mother was still in the hospital.

Women who scored higher than 9 on the EPDS at 8 or 32 weeks postpartum were identified as probable depression cases and were further evaluated using the Spanish language version of the Diagnostic Interview for Genetics Studies (DIGS) (Roca et al., 2007), which was adapted (Sanjuan et al., 2008) to assess the DSM IV criteria for PPD and thereby confirm the diagnosis.

To assess personality traits, the Spanish validated version of the Eysenck Personality Questionnaire-R short scale (EPQ-RS) (Ortet G, 1997) was used. The EPQ-RS consists of 48 items taken from the 100-item EPQ-R and measures the following dimensions of personality: extraversion, neuroticism and psychoticism. We obtained t-scores for the population according to gender and age.

### 2.3 Statistical analysis

Qualitative variables were presented as percentages, and quantitative variables, including maternal age and dimensional personality traits, were presented as means and standard deviations (SD). A chi-square test was used to compare the distribution of categorical qualitative variables across PPD and non-PPD subgroups with the critical value of the residuals of the contingency tables to determine if the observed frequency in a category was higher or lower than expected. The same procedure was used to compare different social variables among occupational status categories. Student's t-test was used to analyze continuous predictor variables, and the McNemar Bowker test was used to compare the frequencies of paired data that indicated differences in occupation status before and during pregnancy. A logistic regression was used to measure the relationship between each of the selected variables (age, marital status, type of coexistence, medical illness, education level, perceived household income and personality traits) and employment status (active versus inactive and sick leave versus other). After identifying occupational status risk factors, we applied a logistic regression to assess a possible association between occupational status during pregnancy and PPD. Marital status, medical illness during pregnancy and maternal personality traits, including neuroticism, psychoticism and extraversion, were included as covariables. Perceived household income was excluded from the logistic regression model because of its colinearity with occupational status during pregnancy, that is, unemployed women had a higher perception of low household income. Education level, although highly associated with occupational status, did not add any significance in the regression models and was therefore excluded in the final analysis. Two multivariate regression models were developed to check our two hypotheses. The first model was applied to assess a possible relationship between sick leave during pregnancy and PPD. The second model was used to assess a possible protective effect of being active, as opposed to being inactive, on PPD. All two-tailed p-values <0.05 were considered to be statistically significant. We used SPSS version 15.0 for all statistical analyses.

## 3. Results

### 3.1 Socio-demographics, obstetric characteristics and personality traits

Of the 1,724 women sampled, 163 (9.5%) were clinically diagnosed as depressed. The socio-demographic, obstetric and maternal personality characteristics are shown in Table 1. Women in the PPD group more frequently lived without a partner (PPD 6.7% versus non-PPD 3.1%; p-value = 0.02), experienced a medical illness during pregnancy (PPD 25.2% versus non-PPD 19.5%; p-value = 0.004) and considered their household income to be low (PPD 46.0% versus non-PPD 35.2%; p-value = 0.001) or very low (PPD 3.1% versus 0.8%; p-value = 0.001). Mothers in the PPD group also recorded higher mean scores for neuroticism (47.2±10.4 versus 40.2±8.2; p-value = 0.001) and psychoticism (47.8±9.1 versus 46.1±8.6; p-value = 0.01) than mothers in the non-PPD group. Conversely, women with PPD had lower mean extraversion scores than women in the non-PPD group (49.0±10.3 versus 51.4±9.6; p-value = 0.001).

### 3.2 Occupation status before and during pregnancy

Figure 1 shows the occupational status before and during pregnancy. Before pregnancy, only 5% of women were inactive, but during pregnancy, this value increased to 23% (Figure 1 panel A). Of those categorized as inactive, 4.4% were unemployed and 0.6% were on sick leave before pregnancy; during pregnancy, 12.2% were unemployed and 10.9% were on sick leave (Figure 1 panel B).

### 3.3 Risk factors for occupation status

Prior to the main analysis, we assessed associations between the socio-demographic, obstetric and personality trait variables and occupation status. Using a binary logistic regression, we explored the association of these variables with being active and being on sick leave (Table 2). Being active was positively associated with a higher level of education (p-value <0.001 for secondary school, and p-value <0.001 for a college degree). We further determined that higher scores for neuroticism and psychoticism were negatively associated with being active (p-value = 0.02 and p-value = 0.01, respectively). Sick leave was associated with a younger age (p-values = 0.004), the presence of a medical illness (p-value = 0.001) and lower levels of education (p-value <0.019 for secondary school and p-value = 0.003 for primary school). While living with parents appeared to protect against sick leave, the result was not statistically significant (p-value = 0.06).

| Variables | Total sample | PPD | Non-PPD | P |
|---|---|---|---|---|
| **Participants (N)** | 1724 | 163 | 1561 | |
| **Age (years)**[a] | 31.8±4.6 | 31.7±5.0 | 31.8±4.6 | 0.85 |
| **Living with partner (%)**[b] | | | | |
| Yes | 96.6 | 93.3 | 96.9 | 0.02 |
| No | 3.4 | 6.7 | 3.1 | |
| **Type of coexistence (%)** | | | | |
| Parents | 3.6 | 3.1 | 3.7 | |
| Own family | 94.7 | 94.5 | 94.7 | 0.72 |
| Other | 1.7 | 2.5 | 1.7 | |
| **Medical illness**[c] | | | | |
| Yes | 16.8 | 25.2 | 15.9 | 0.004 |
| No | 83.2 | 74.8 | 84.1 | |
| **Education level (%)** | | | | |
| Primary school | 30.5 | 33.7 | 30.2 | |
| Secondary school | 41.4 | 42.3 | 41.3 | 0.42 |
| College degree | 28.1 | 23.9 | 28.5 | |
| **Perceived household income (%)** | | | | |
| Adequate | 62.8 | 50.9 | 64.1 | |
| Low | 36.2 | 46.0 | 35.2 | <0.001 |
| Very low | 1.0 | 3.1 | 0.8 | |
| **Personality traits**[a] | | | | |
| Extraversion | 51.2±9.1 | 49.0±10.3 | 51.4±9.0 | 0.001 |
| Neuroticism | 40.9±8.6 | 47.2±10.4 | 40.24±8.2 | 0.0001 |
| Psychoticism | 46.2±8.6 | 47.8±9.1 | 46.1±8.6 | 0.01 |

[a]Values are given as mean ±SD and compared to student's t-test
[b]Values are given as percentages and compared by chi-square test
[c]Includes any medical condition that involved either hospitalization or pharmacological treatment during pregnancy and immediately before, during or after delivery

Table 1. Socio-demographic, obstetric and personality trait variables for all participants and for the PPD and non-PPD groups.

### 3.4 Occupational status and PPD

Figure 2 shows the percentages of active and inactive women before and during pregnancy. The percentages of active (95%) and inactive (5%) women before pregnancy were similar in the group of women who developed PPD compared with the group that did not develop PPD (Figure 2 panel A). During pregnancy, however, the percentage of inactive women increased from 5% to 22% in the group that did not develop PPD and from 5% to 36% in the

| | Active vs. Inactive[a] | | | Sick leave vs. Active | | |
|---|---|---|---|---|---|---|
| **Variables** | **OR[b]** | **CI** | **P** | **OR** | **CI** | **P** |
| **Age** | 0.98 | 0.96 – 1.01 | 0.30 | 1.05 | 1.01 – 1.08 | 0.004 |
| **Living with partner (%)** | | | | | | |
| Yes | 1.00 | | | 1.00 | | |
| No | 0.67 | 0.33 – 1.33 | 0.25 | 0.42 | 0.13 – 1.37 | 0.15 |
| **Type of coexistence (%)** | | | | | | |
| Own family | 1.00 | | | 1.00 | | |
| Parents | 0.55 | 0.27 – 1.13 | 0.10 | 0.25 | 0.06 – 1.05 | 0.06 |
| Other | 0.81 | 0.33 - 2.01 | 0.65 | 0.28 | 0.03 – 2.09 | 0.21 |
| **Medical ilnesss[c]** | | | | | | |
| No | 1.00 | | | 1.00 | | |
| Yes | 1.23 | 0.92 – 1.64 | 0.15 | 1.79 | 1.25 – 2.56 | 0.001 |
| **Education level (%)** | | | | | | |
| College degree | 1.00 | | | 1.00 | | |
| Secondary school | 1.75 | 1.28 – 2.38 | <0.001 | 1.61 | 1.08 – 2.41 | 0.019 |
| Primary school | 2.70 | 1.97 – 3.69 | <0.001 | 1.91 | 1.25 – 2.91 | 0.003 |
| **Perceived household income (%)** | | | | | | |
| Adequate | 1.00 | | | 1.00 | | |
| Low | 1.28 | 1.02 – 1.62 | 0.03 | 1.02 | 0.74 – 1.41 | 0.86 |
| Very low | 1.12 | 0.36 – 3.49 | 0.83 | 0.54 | 0.07 – 4.20 | 0.56 |
| **Personality traits** | | | | | | |
| Extraversion | 1.00 | 0.99 – 1.02 | 0.21 | 1.00 | 0.98 – 1.02 | 0.45 |
| Neuroticism | 1.01 | 1.00 – 1.02 | 0.02 | 1.01 | 0.99 – 1.03 | 0.17 |
| Psychoticism | 1.02 | 1.00 – 1.03 | 0.01 | 1.01 | 0.99 – 1.03 | 0.15 |

[a]Active defined as employed, housewife or student and inactive as unemployed and on sick leave
[b]Binary logistic regression
[c]Includes any medical condition that involved either hospitalization or pharmacological treatment during pregnancy and immediately before, during or after delivery

Table 2. Odds ratios (ORs) and 95% confidence intervals (CIs) for occupational status in relation to selected socioeconomic, obstetric and personality trait variables for 1,724 Spanish participants.

group that did. The increase in inactivity status during pregnancy was due to an increase in unemployment, from 4.5% to 11.9% in the non-PPD group and from 4.3% to 15.3% in the PPD group, and an increase in sick leave, from 0.6% to 9.9% in the non-PPD group and from 0.6% to 20.9% in the PPD group. Inactivity before pregnancy was not associated with PPD (data not shown); however, inactivity during pregnancy was statistically different in the PPD group compared with the non-PPD group (Figure 3).

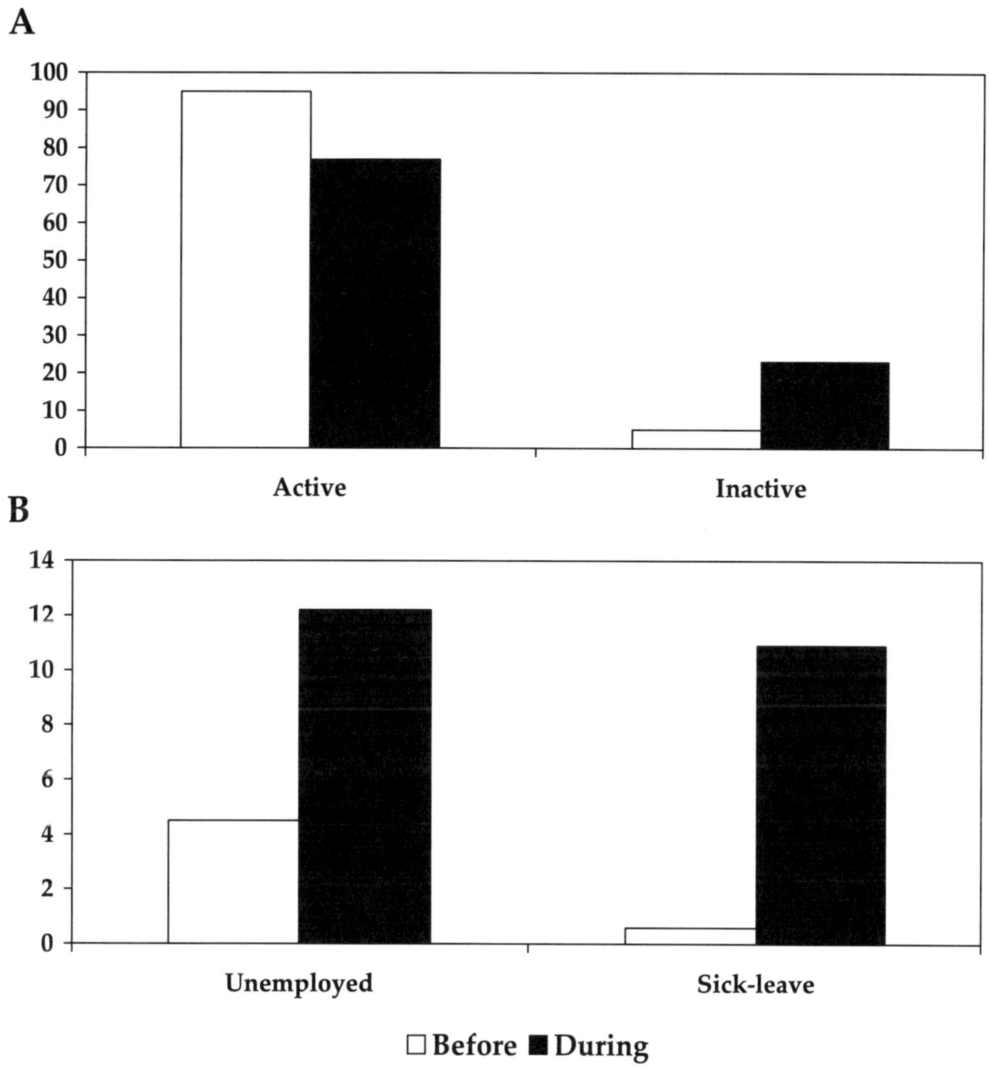


Fig. 1. **Occupation status before and during pregnancy.**
Panel A shows the distribution of women according to their occupation status of active (employed, student or housewife) or inactive (unemployed or on sick leave). Panel B shows the distribution of inactive women according to their status of unemployed or on sick leave. Open bars represent values before pregnancy, and filled bars represent values during pregnancy. MacNemar Bowker test p-value $<0.001$.

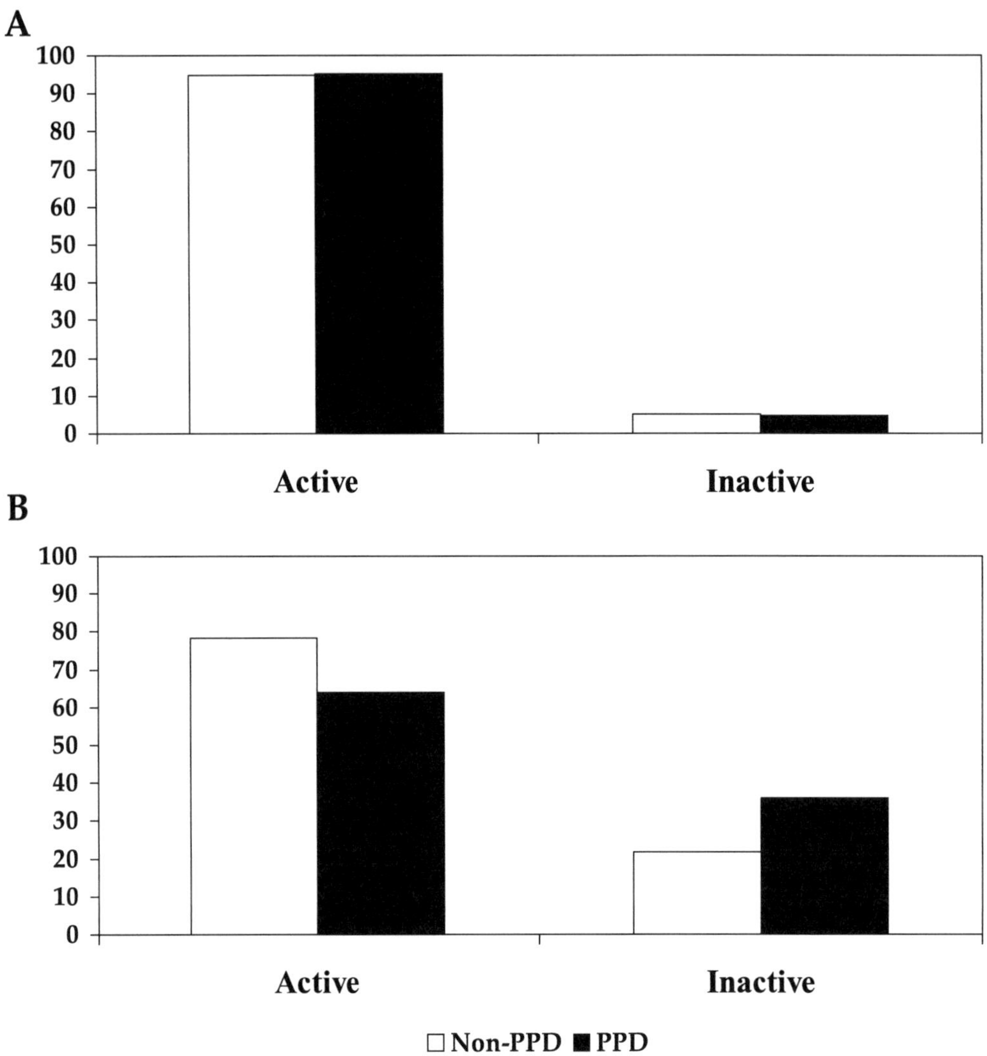


Fig. 2. **Occupation status before and during pregnancy and PPD.**
Panel A shows the distribution of active and inactive women before pregnancy according to the diagnosed presence or absence of PPD. Panel B shows the distribution of active and inactive women during pregnancy according to their PPD diagnosis. Open bars represent women who did not develop PPD, and filled bars represent women who did develop PPD. MacNemar Bowker test p=value <0.001.

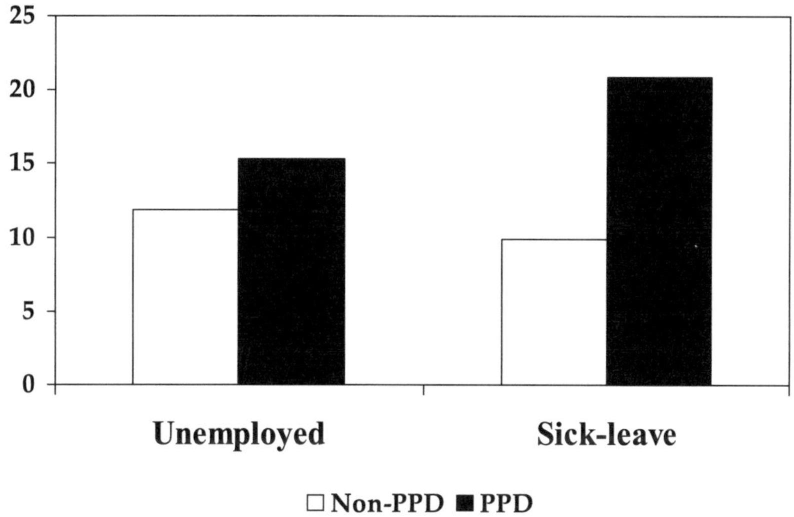


Fig. 3. **Inactivity during pregnancy and PPD.**
The distribution of women categorized as inactive (unemployed or on sick leave) during pregnancy, according to their subsequent PPD diagnoses. Open bars represent women who did not develop PPD, and filled bars represent women who did develop PPD. ANOVA p-value <0.001.

Finally, using a multivariate logistic regression analysis, we explored the relationship between occupation status and PPD, considering personality traits as covariables. The socio-demographic and obstetric variables explored in the binary logistic regression were included as covariables. Two models were constructed; one explored the risk that being on sick leave will lead to PPD, and the other explored the way in which being active protects against PPD. These results are shown in Table 3.

In summary, being on sick leave, not having a partner, having a medical illness and demonstrating a likelihood for neuroticism are all indicators of risk for PPD. The multivariate model explains 13% of the PPD variance (Nagelkerke $R^2$ = 0.135). While the variable "being on sick leave" is an independent risk factor for PPD, its strong correlation with the variable "presence of medical illness" is noteworthy. Being active, having a partner and not having a medical illness appear to prevent the development of PPD. The model also explains 13% of the PPD variance.

| Regression model | Variables in the equation | Wald statistic | β | OR (95% CI) | P |
|---|---|---|---|---|---|
| **Model 1. Sick-leave risk to PPD[a]** | | | | | |
| | Living without partner | 6.36 | 0.94 | 2.56 (1.23-5.34) | 0.012 |
| | Presence of medical illness | 4.36 | 0.43 | 1.54 (1.02-2.31) | 0.037 |
| | Being on sick leave | 19.09 | 0.98 | 2.68 (1.72-4.18) | 0.0001 |
| | Unemployed | 2.56 | 0.397 | 1.48 (0.91-2.41) | 0.109 |
| | Extraversion | 2.60 | -0.014 | 0.98 (0.98-1.00) | 0.10 |
| | Neuroticism | 63.57 | 0.075 | 1.07 (1.05-1.09) | 0.0001 |
| | Psychoticism | 0.072 | -0.003 | 0.99 (0.97-1.01) | 0.78 |
| **Model 2. Being active protection to PPD[b]** | | | | | |
| | Living with partner | 6.0 | -0.91 | 0.40 (0.19-0.83) | 0.014 |
| | Absence of medical illness | 5.1 | -0.46 | 0.62 (0.42-0.94) | 0.024 |
| | Active occupational status | 14.7 | -0.70 | 0.50 (0.35-0.70) | <0.001 |
| | Extraversion | 2.5 | -0.014 | 0.99 (0.97-1.00) | 0.11 |
| | Neuroticism | 62.2 | 0.074 | 1.07 (1.05-1.09) | <0.001 |
| | Psychoticism | 0.09 | -0.003 | 0.99 (0.98-1.01) | 0.75 |

[a]The "enter" method was used. Hosmer-Lemeshow $P=0.81$. Nagelkerke $R^2= 0.13$
[b]The "enter" method was used. Hosmer-Lemeshow $P=0.55$. Nagelkerke $R^2= 0.13$

Table 3. Multivariate logistic regression analysis to assess the relationship between occupational status and PPD.

## 4. Discussion

PPD was identified in 9.5% of subjects, in agreement with PPD prevalences in other studies (O'Hara, 2009). The percentage of women categorized as inactive before pregnancy was 4.5% lower than the official percentage of unemployment during the period of our study in Spain (2003-2004; National Institute of Statistics) in an age- and gender-match comparison. Note that data from the National Institute of Statistics refers exclusively to employment, and we included in the activity group employed women but also students and housewife activity. Surprisingly, the percentage of inactive women increased to 23% during pregnancy. An important cause for this dramatic change was the increase in sick leave, which increased 18 times over the normal rate of women on sick leave. However, research has indicated that sick-leave frequency increases during pregnancy (Josefsson et al., 2002; A. Sydsjo et al., 2001). Interestingly, unemployment during pregnancy in our sample almost tripled. Because we excluded women with depression during pregnancy, this increase in sick leave was not likely caused by depression, as other authors have reported (Bermejo et al., 2010). As we did not collect evidence regarding the cause of this increase, we do not know if pregnant women decided not to work or if their unemployment was due to employee discrimination. The strong association among a low level of education, sick leave and unemployment suggest that women with lower levels of education have discontinuous jobs that, perhaps by one's own decision, are not renewed following pregnancy.

On the basis of previous reports (Akman, Uguz, & Kaya, 2007; Beck, 2001), we hypothesized that neuroticism would strongly influence occupation status and, consequently, the development of PPD. Our binary logistic regression results show that neuroticism and psychoticism were significantly associated with an inactive occupation status, albeit with a very low OR (OR = 1.01 and 1.02, respectively). Because the inactive category included unemployment and sick leave, we explored the association of neuroticism with unemployment and sick leave separately and identified an association with unemployment but not with sick leave. Pregnant women with higher neuroticism scores are potentially more likely to be unemployed because of their perception of poor personal health (Alfonsi et al., 2011). Surprisingly, however, a significant number of women with high psychoticism scores were unemployed. This could be because women with higher psychoticism scores have significant social disabilities and are thus unable to find jobs. A higher level of education was associated with a better occupation status, possibly because a better education makes finding a job easier.

The most important finding is that being on sick leave tripled the risk for PPD. This risk was heightened for those living without a partner, having higher scores for neuroticism and having a medical illness during pregnancy. Neuroticism and the presence of a medical illness are independent risk factors for PPD; thus, their statistical significance in the model was maintained in the multivariate analysis. We also found that being active reduced the risk of PPD by one half. This protection from PPD increased when a woman was living with a partner, had no medical illness during pregnancy and had lower neuroticism scores. Our model of risk variables for the link between occupation status and PPD is summarized in Figure 4. Previous studies have reported an association between maternal neuroticism and PPD (Jones et al., 2010) while others have studied the association between socioeconomic factors and PPD (Akincigil, Munch, & Niemczyk, 2010). However, no studies have examined the relationship among a mother's personality traits, socioeconomic variables and PPD.

Sickness is associated with a compromised level of health in non-pregnant women (Bermejo et al., 2010), and the accompanying lowered self-perception often results in a decreased level of physical activity. The main reason for sick leave during pregnancy is back pain (G. Sydsjo & Sydsjo, 2005). Previous reports have indicated that physical activity during pregnancy plays an important role in minimizing the risk of PPD (Ersek & Brunner Huber, 2009). Sick leave may be associated with adverse social and economic consequences, both of which have been implicated in PPD (Boyd, Mogul, Newman, & Coyne, 2011). Our results are consistent with previous studies that show employment, especially full-time, and a professional or technical job during pregnancy may reduce the risk of PPD (Inandi et al., 2002; Jardri et al., 2006; Lane et al., 1997; Miyake et al., 2011; Rubertsson et al., 2005; Warner et al., 1996). However, some researchers did not find an association between employment and PPD (Akman et al., 2007; Ekuklu, Tokuc, Eskiocak, Berberoglu, & Saltik, 2004; Goyal, Gay, & Lee, 2010; Rich-Edwards et al., 2006; Tannous, Gigante, Fuchs, & Busnello, 2008; Weiss, Sheehan, & Gushwa, 2009). This controversy can be partially explained by several methodological differences in the studies.

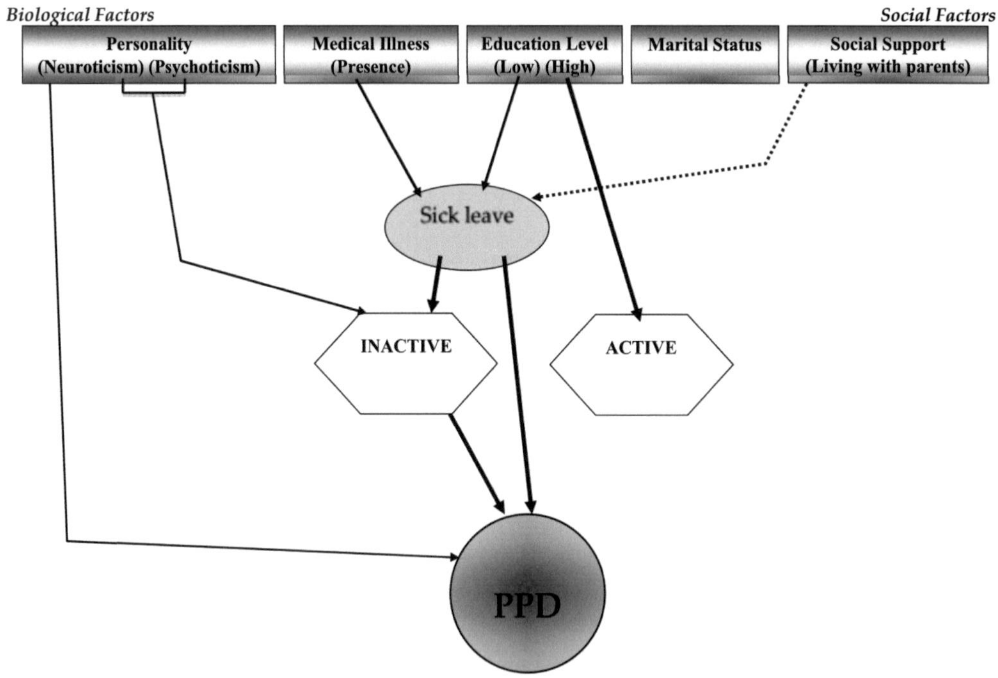


Fig. 4. **The direct or indirect relationship between selected variables and PPD.** Thickness of lines is proportional to p-value. Discontinuous lines represent a non-significant association (p-value = 0.06).

Our study had several methodological strengths. The sample size of 1,724 is large, and the sample group was composed exclusively of Spanish Caucasian women. The presence of a psychiatric illness during pregnancy was an exclusion criteria; thus, biases due to psychiatric conditions were avoided. Although previous studies have assessed employment during pregnancy and PPD, to our knowledge, this is the first study to assess the association of criteria other than employment status with PPD. Moreover, we used a psychiatric diagnostic of PPD based on the DSM IV that considers a broad period of occurrence. Most studies have been based only on the presence of depressive symptoms. Finally, our study explored the relationship between occupation and PPD while also considering individual neuroticism scores.

However, our study also has limitations. Some interesting variables such as the cause of sick leave, the level of marital quality support, an accurate diagnostic of illness during pregnancy and job type were not registered because this study was initially designed to explore a genetic-environment vulnerability to PPD (Sanjuan et al., 2008). Despite its limitations and the need for future investigations, interesting insights can be drawn from this work. First, sick leave may not produce the intended benefits expected by pregnant women. Pregnancy is associated with asthenia, back pain and insomnia. As a result, family doctors and obstetricians often grant sick leave without a clear medical cause to avoid conflicts (Larsson, Sydsjo, Alexanderson, & Sydsjo, 2006). Perhaps a more reflexive attitude is to implement psycho-educational interventions for pregnant women in an attempt to reduce unnecessary sick leave requests. For instance, for cases in which a medical condition requires a sick leave, other activities should be programmed to maintain a certain level of physical activity and self-esteem. We believe that if information regarding marital status, occupation status and maternal personality traits were collected and included in the obstetric history, identifying women who are at a high risk of developing PPD would be easier. This low-cost and relatively easy solution would assist in postpartum follow-up examinations of women with an increased susceptibility to PPD. Intervention studies to support this conclusion should be conducted.

## 5. References

Akincigil, A., Munch, S., & Niemczyk, K. C. (2010). Predictors of maternal depression in the first year postpartum: Marital status and mediating role of relationship quality. *Social Work in Health Care, 49*(3), 227-244.

Akman, C., Uguz, F., & Kaya, N. (2007). Postpartum-onset major depression is associated with personality disorders. *Comprehensive Psychiatry, 48*(4), 343-347.

Albacar, G., Sans, T., Martin-Santos, R., Garcia-Esteve, L., Guillamat, R., Sanjuan, J., et al. (2011). An association between plasma ferritin concentrations measured 48 h after delivery and postpartum depression. *Journal of Affective Disorders, 131*(1-3), 136-142.

Alfonsi, G., Conway, M., & Pushkar, D. (2011). The lower subjective social status of neurotic individuals: Multiple pathways through occupational prestige, income, and illness. *Journal of Personality, 79*(3), 619-642.

Beck, C. T. (2001). Predictors of postpartum depression: An update. *Nursing Research, 50*(5), 275-285.

Bermejo, I., Kriston, L., Schneider, F., Gaebel, W., Hegerl, U., Berger, M., et al. (2010). Sick leave and depression - determining factors and clinical effect in outpatient care. *Psychiatry Research, 180*(2-3), 68-73.

Boyd, R. C., Mogul, M., Newman, D., & Coyne, J. C. (2011). Screening and referral for postpartum depression among low-income women: A qualitative perspective from community health workers. *Depression Research and Treatment, 2011*, 320605.

Brummelte, S., & Galea, L. A. (2010). Depression during pregnancy and postpartum: Contribution of stress and ovarian hormones. *Progress in Neuro-Psychopharmacology & Biological Psychiatry, 34*(5), 766-776.

Chen, C. H. (2001). Association of work status and mental well-being in new mothers. *The Kaohsiung Journal of Medical Sciences, 17*(11), 570-575.

Costas, J., Gratacos, M., Escaramis, G., Martin-Santos, R., de Diego, Y., Baca-Garcia, E., et al. (2010). Association study of 44 candidate genes with depressive and anxiety symptoms in post-partum women. *Journal of Psychiatric Research, 44*(11), 717-724.

Ekuklu, G., Tokuc, B., Eskiocak, M., Berberoglu, U., & Saltik, A. (2004). Prevalence of postpartum depression in edirne, turkey, and related factors. *The Journal of Reproductive Medicine, 49*(11), 908-914.

Ersek, J. L., & Brunner Huber, L. R. (2009). Physical activity prior to and during pregnancy and risk of postpartum depressive symptoms. *Journal of Obstetric, Gynecologic, and Neonatal Nursing : JOGNN / NAACOG, 38*(5), 556-566.

Garcia-Esteve, L., Ascaso, C., Ojuel, J., & Navarro, P. (2003). Validation of the edinburgh postnatal depression scale (EPDS) in spanish mothers. *Journal of Affective Disorders, 75*(1), 71-76.

Goyal, D., Gay, C., & Lee, K. A. (2010). How much does low socioeconomic status increase the risk of prenatal and postpartum depressive symptoms in first-time mothers? *Women's Health Issues : Official Publication of the Jacobs Institute of Women's Health, 20*(2), 96-104.

Inandi, T., Elci, O. C., Ozturk, A., Egri, M., Polat, A., & Sahin, T. K. (2002). Risk factors for depression in postnatal first year, in eastern turkey. *International Journal of Epidemiology, 31*(6), 1201-1207.

Jardri, R., Pelta, J., Maron, M., Thomas, P., Delion, P., Codaccioni, X., et al. (2006). Predictive validation study of the edinburgh postnatal depression scale in the first week after delivery and risk analysis for postnatal depression. *Journal of Affective Disorders, 93*(1-3), 169-176.

Jones, L., Scott, J., Cooper, C., Forty, L., Smith, K. G., Sham, P., et al. (2010). Cognitive style, personality and vulnerability to postnatal depression. *The British Journal of Psychiatry : The Journal of Mental Science, 196*(3), 200-205.

Josefsson, A., Angelsioo, L., Berg, G., Ekstrom, C. M., Gunnervik, C., Nordin, C., et al. (2002). Obstetric, somatic, and demographic risk factors for postpartum depressive symptoms. *Obstetrics and Gynecology, 99*(2), 223-228.

Kozinszky, Z., Dudas, R. B., Csatordai, S., Devosa, I., Toth, E., Szabo, D., et al. (2011). Social dynamics of postpartum depression: A population-based screening in south-eastern hungary. *Social Psychiatry and Psychiatric Epidemiology, 46*(5), 413-423.

Lane, A., Keville, R., Morris, M., Kinsella, A., Turner, M., & Barry, S. (1997). Postnatal depression and elation among mothers and their partners: Prevalence and predictors. *The British Journal of Psychiatry : The Journal of Mental Science, 171*, 550-555.

Larsson, C., Sydsjo, A., Alexanderson, K., & Sydsjo, G. (2006). Obstetricians' attitudes and opinions on sickness absence and benefits during pregnancy. *Acta Obstetricia Et Gynecologica Scandinavica, 85*(2), 165-170.

Leung, B. M., & Kaplan, B. J. (2009). Perinatal depression: Prevalence, risks, and the nutrition link--a review of the literature. *Journal of the American Dietetic Association, 109*(9), 1566-1575.

Mahon, P. B., Payne, J. L., MacKinnon, D. F., Mondimore, F. M., Goes, F. S., Schweizer, B., et al. (2009). Genome-wide linkage and follow-up association study of postpartum mood symptoms. *The American Journal of Psychiatry, 166*(11), 1229-1237.

McGarry, J., Kim, H., Sheng, X., Egger, M., & Baksh, L. (2009). Postpartum depression and help-seeking behavior. *Journal of Midwifery & Women's Health, 54*(1), 50-56.

Miyake, Y., Tanaka, K., Sasaki, S., & Hirota, Y. (2011). Employment, income, and education and risk of postpartum depression: The osaka maternal and child health study. *Journal of Affective Disorders, 130*(1-2), 133-137.

O'Hara, M. W. (2009). Postpartum depression: What we know. *Journal of Clinical Psychology, 65*(12), 1258-1269.

Oppo, A., Mauri, M., Ramacciotti, D., Camilleri, V., Banti, S., Borri, C., et al. (2009). Risk factors for postpartum depression: The role of the postpartum depression predictors inventory-revised (PDPI-R). results from the perinatal depression-research & screening unit (PNDReScU) study. *Archives of Women's Mental Health, 12*(4), 239-249.

Ortet G, M. M. (1997). *Cuestionario revisado de personalidad Eysenk*. Madrid: TEA Ediciones SA.

Pearlstein, T., Howard, M., Salisbury, A., & Zlotnick, C. (2009). Postpartum depression. *American Journal of Obstetrics and Gynecology, 200*(4), 357-364.

Posmontier, B. (2008). Functional status outcomes in mothers with and without postpartum depression. *Journal of Midwifery & Women's Health, 53*(4), 310-318.

Rich-Edwards, J. W., Kleinman, K., Abrams, A., Harlow, B. L., McLaughlin, T. J., Joffe, H., et al. (2006). Sociodemographic predictors of antenatal and postpartum depressive symptoms among women in a medical group practice. *Journal of Epidemiology and Community Health, 60*(3), 221-227.

Roca, M., Martin-Santos, R., Saiz, J., Obiols, J., Serrano, M. J., Torrens, M., et al. (2007). Diagnostic interview for genetic studies (DIGS): Inter-rater and test-retest reliability and validity in a spanish population. *European Psychiatry : The Journal of the Association of European Psychiatrists, 22*(1), 44-48.

Rubertsson, C., Wickberg, B., Gustavsson, P., & Radestad, I. (2005). Depressive symptoms in early pregnancy, two months and one year postpartum-prevalence and psychosocial risk factors in a national swedish sample. *Archives of Women's Mental Health, 8*(2), 97-104.

Sanjuan, J., Martin-Santos, R., Garcia-Esteve, L., Carot, J. M., Guillamat, R., Gutierrez-Zotes, A., et al. (2008). Mood changes after delivery: Role of the serotonin transporter gene. *The British Journal of Psychiatry : The Journal of Mental Science, 193*(5), 383-388.

Stankunas, M., Kalediene, R., Starkuviene, S., & Kapustinskiene, V. (2006). Duration of unemployment and depression: A cross-sectional survey in lithuania. *BMC Public Health, 6*, 174.

Sydsjo, A., Sydsjo, G., & Alexanderson, K. (2001). Influence of pregnancy-related diagnoses on sick-leave data in women aged 16-44. *Journal of Women's Health & Gender-Based Medicine, 10*(7), 707-714.

Sydsjo, G., & Sydsjo, A. (2005). No association found between sickness absence and duration of pregnancy benefit. *Scandinavian Journal of Primary Health Care, 23*(3), 178-183.

Tannous, L., Gigante, L. P., Fuchs, S. C., & Busnello, E. D. (2008). Postnatal depression in southern brazil: Prevalence and its demographic and socioeconomic determinants. *BMC Psychiatry, 8*, 1.

Treloar, S. A., Martin, N. G., Bucholz, K. K., Madden, P. A., & Heath, A. C. (1999). Genetic influences on post-natal depressive symptoms: Findings from an australian twin sample. *Psychological Medicine, 29*(3), 645-654.

Warner, R., Appleby, L., Whitton, A., & Faragher, B. (1996). Demographic and obstetric risk factors for postnatal psychiatric morbidity. *The British Journal of Psychiatry : The Journal of Mental Science, 168*(5), 607-611.

Weiss, B. D., Sheehan, C. P., & Gushwa, L. L. (2009). Is low literacy a risk factor for symptoms of depression in postpartum women? *The Journal of Reproductive Medicine*, *54*(9), 563-568.

# 6

# Postnatal Depression and Emotion: The Misfortune of Mother-Infant Interactions

Sandrine Gil[1], Sylvie Droit-Volet[2],
Virginie Laval[1] and Frédérique Teissèdre[2]
[1]*Centre de Recherches sur la Cognition et l'Apprentissage (CeRCA – UMR6234) – University of Poitiers*
[2]*Laboratoire de Psychologie Sociale et Cognitive (LAPSCO – UMR6024) University of Clermont – Ferrand - France*

## 1. Introduction

*"The movements of expression in the face and body (…) serve as the first means of communication between the mother and her child; she smiles approval, and thus encourages her child on the right path, or frowns disapproval"* Charles Darwin (1872/1998, p. 359).

Emotional communication can be viewed as a fundamental factor in children's emotional, social, and cognitive development. Most developmental psychologists agree that the recognition and expression of emotions through early social interaction between the mother and the child play a particularly important role in children's development (Bandura, 1992; Bowlby, 1969; Sroufe, 1996; Trevarthen, 1979). Moreover, as Paul Ekman reminds us, nature and nurture are both intrinsically involved in children's psychological development: *"It is never a question only of nature or only of nurture. We are biosocial creatures, our minds are embodied, reflecting our lives and the lives of our ancestors."* Ekman (1996, p. 393). This biosocial conception of emotional development, defended in the theories put forward by a number of pioneers in the child development field, therefore suggests that the child-caregiver relation constitutes a system which is simultaneously based on the innate skills of the baby while also having the task of elaborating and refining these skills.

As of the first months of life, emotional and social development is grounded in emotional communication, i.e. in a social environment which forms or modulates primary abilities (Izard, 1971; Sroufe, 1979). Therefore, the mother-infant interaction constitutes the first and main environmental context that might shape infants' abilities. Before the development of language in the child, mother-child communication is largely non-verbal. It is based on a whole range of non-verbal signals (e.g. facial expression, prosody, touch) produced by the mother. Numerous studies have shown that the quality of these different non-verbal signals is impaired in mothers suffering from postpartum depression. The question is: what are the effects of an early impairment of communication on children's development?

The aim of this chapter is therefore to review the literature relating to psychological studies of mothers suffering from depression and the impact of their depression on early mother-child relationships. The originality of our contribution lies in the fact that it focuses on emotion, i.e. the emotional regulation and dysregulation themselves, as well as on their causes and consequences for both the mother and for the socio-emotional development of her baby.

## 2. An early ability to process emotion in infants: The mother as the preferred object of processing

A large body of literature has revealed that, from birth onwards, human babies are equipped with wide-ranging, deeply innate mechanism which serve an adaptive function. These biological mechanisms are thought to help human beings deal with their physical and social environments and thus contribute to both their survival and their well-being (Darwin, 1872/1998; Ekman, 1982; Izard & Malatesta, 1987; Leslie, 1987). As Trevarthen (1998) argues, newborns have innate intersubjectivity: *"The claim made, while not questioning that development involves learning or that infants depend on care, underlined that a child is born with motives to find and use the motives of other persons in 'conversational' negotiation of purposes, emotions, experiences and meaning."* (Trevarthen, 1998, p. 16). Such pre-adaptation for emotional communication in infants has been demonstrated by a number of well-known face discrimination studies that have described how neonates are extremely sensitive to human faces, how they respond selectively to them, and how they imitate emotions perceived in adults. In these studies, researchers presented neonates with a series of stimuli that represented human faces, non-human face-like patterns, or scrambled patterns (Figure 1). They then measured whether the neonates preferentially directed their gaze, or looked longer, at any one specific type of stimulus. They found that neonates, who have a minimal experience of faces, prefer human face-like patterns (Goren et al., 1975; Johnson et al., 1991; Mondloch et al., 1999). Using the same procedure, Batki et al. (2000) showed that neonates prefer to orient their attention toward faces which have open eyes (Batki et al., 2000). These studies therefore indicate that babies are innately interested in processing human faces.

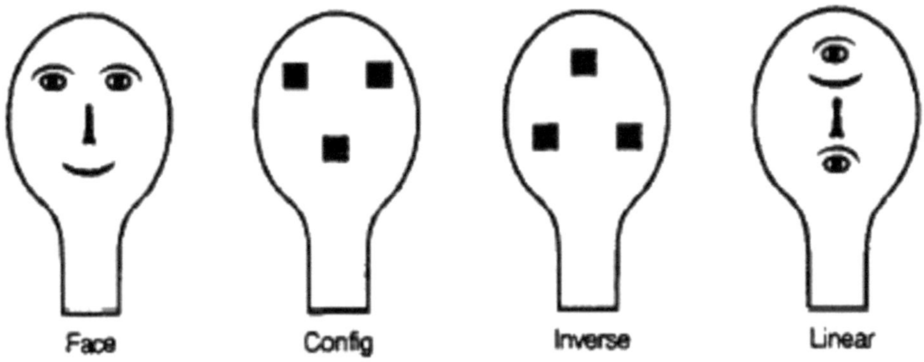


Fig. 1. Examples of face-related stimuli used to demonstrate the face-preference of babies. Source: Johnson et al. (1991).

In 1977, Meltzoff and Moore showed that neonates not only preferentially focus their attention on faces, but that they are also able to imitate the facial expressions perceived on those faces. From two to three weeks of life, when adults stick out their tongues, form a kiss with their lips, or open their mouth, infants imitate these facial expressions (see Figure 2).

There is also ample evidence that newborns are able to express some adult-like emotional facial patterns in response to emotion elicitors (Camras et al., 1991; Rosenstein & Oster, 1988). As of an early age starting shortly after birth, babies are therefore able to process other people's facial expressions, especially those of the mother, and embody other people's emotions through imitation.

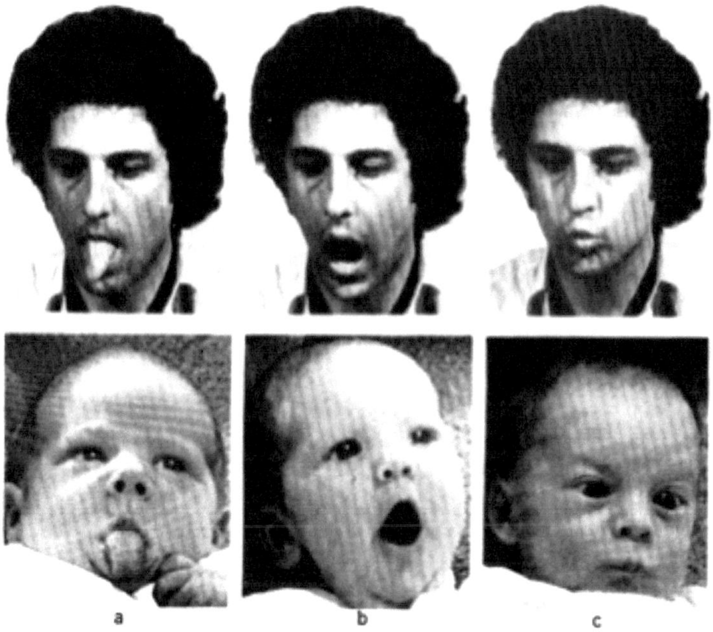


Fig. 2. Sample photographs taken from videos of infants imitating an adult experimenter (a: tongue protrusion; b: mouth opening; c: lip protrusion). Source: Meltzoff & Moore (1977).

The fact that infants possess early emotional communication abilities is now a well-established psychological fact. As a result, researchers are agreed in considering that children's socio-emotional development may be shaped by their socio-emotional environment, and more particularly by their initial experiences during a period of life that is critical for the establishment of abilities. More precisely, it is now widely believed that the infant's ability to express and recognize affective states can be shaped by early interactions. The study conducted by Pascalis and his team (2002) clearly revealed the critical role of experience in the shaping of infant's face processing abilities. In their jolly study, they examined the ability of infants to discriminate between the identities of faces as a function of their experience of human faces. They presented pairs of human faces or monkey faces to infants of different ages. Their results showed that the infants were able to discriminate equally between two different identities in the two species at the age of 6 months, whereas they were able to do it only for human faces at the age of 9 months (Pascalis et al., 2002). Experience of human faces therefore leads to a sort of specialization in the processing of human faces. This is referred to as "perceptual narrowing" and clearly indicates the considerable impact of experience on the development of early social abilities.

Interactions between babies and their mothers represent the majority of the emotional interactions experienced by infants and thus constitute the primary environment for emotional learning (Papousek & Papousek, 1989; Tronick, 1989). Consequently, it may be assumed that non-verbal communication, for example in the form of emotional facial expressions, plays a critical role in the establishment of early social interaction and the development of social abilities. Facial expressions are indeed the main way in which two partners are able to interact and develop an intimate relationship, and in which mothers can understand their infants and respond to their needs. In line with the "intuitive parenting" concept, (Papousek & Papousek, 1978), Schoetzau and Papousek (1977) illustrated how face-to-face contact is an essential part of the communication between the mother and her baby. Indeed, these authors showed that mothers watch their babies sleeping at a distance of 40-50 cm, but that as soon as their infants open their eyes, they immediately reduce the face-to-face distance and position their faces in the middle of the infant's visual field. The postpartum period is thus a critical period during which links are established between the mother and her baby. However, this very special moment can be disrupted by a series of emotional and psychiatric disorders that can be experienced by mothers.

## 3. Risks of an early infant-mother interaction disrupted by the depression of the mother

The likelihood of mothers being admitted into a psychiatric unit appears to be multiplied by a factor of between 10 and 20 during the first month following delivery. After giving birth, mothers may present a variety of emotional disorders such as stress, anxiety and depression that vary in their severity and time of onset. Anxiety, stress and postpartum blues are generally short-lived. Postpartum blues takes the form of emotional disturbances such as crying, anxiety, and a depressed and unstable mood. It is thought to affect a non-negligible proportion of mothers, which varies from 20 to 80 % depending on the study. This disrupted emotional state can be observed during the first 15 days following the birth. It is in fact considered to be a premature form of postpartum depression. Indeed, numerous studies have shown that an intense and prolonged period of postpartum blues could represent the onset of postpartum depression. This latter condition can last for several months and affects 10 to 20 % of women who have just given birth (Beck, 2002). Moreover, the link between blues and depression has been documented on the basis of the Edinburg Postnatal Depression Scale (EPDS) that is thought to evaluate the depressive component of postpartum blues and to predict the clinical diagnosis of postpartum depression (Chabrol & Teissèdre, 2004; Gonidakis et al., 2008). More rarely, mothers can also exhibit more serious disorders such as puerperal psychosis (1-2 per thousand deliveries). This dramatic state occurs within the first 2-4 weeks after delivery and is characterized by paranoid, delusions, confused cognitive manifestations, and a significant level of disorganized behavior (Sit et al., 2006). The symptoms of a depressive state are thus difficult for mothers to cope with, particularly during a period of their lives when they must both cope with a newborn child who is dependent upon them and adhere to the role of good mother as expected by their families and society. Moreover, as we will explain below, these depressive symptoms can lead to non-optimal early mother-child interactions, due to both a characteristic depressive style of emotional expressiveness and the way in which emotional cues are processed. As stated by de Haan et al. (2004, p. 1214), because *"linkages detected between maternal emotional disposition and infant face processing reflect, at least in part, the role of experience in shaping face processing,"* examining the behavior of depressed mothers during the first months of their babies' lives is a valuable way of gaining an understanding of their effect on children's socio-emotional development within the context of an early undertaking to care for the child.

Among the emotional behaviors, facial expressions play a crucial role in communication. As Ursula Hess (2001) stresses, facial expressions are important not only for the person who displays them, but also for the perceiver who has to associate them with a meaning in order to react appropriately (Keltner & Haidt, 2001; Frijda, 2007; Russell & Fernandez-Dols, 1997). In the case of depression, the predominant facial expression is that of sadness. As an emotion, sadness is an occasional phenomenon. However, in the case of depression, it is more like a mood, the affective component of emotions. Whereas emotions color life at a specific time, a mood fundamentally colors every part of our lives. It is therefore a continuous emotional state. According to the DSM IV criteria (American Psychiatry Association, 1994), sadness is a characteristic of a depressive mood. In this case, sadness is pathological because it is excessive, maladaptive, persistent and aggravated. More specifically, this pathological sad mood is a common criterion in the diagnosis of major depression and postpartum depression, the latter being considered as a special case of the former, although it is necessary to differentiate between them in terms of etiology and treatment (see Hendrick et al., 2000).

However, few studies have investigated the specificity of atypical emotional behavior in mothers with depressive symptoms after birth compared to women with major depression. In addition, it is not always easy to identify how major depression and postpartum depression have been differentiated in the studies published to date. This raises several questions concerning the etiology of depressive symptoms: Are women diagnosed as depressed because of their postpartum state or because it is the first time they have been screened for depression? Whatever the case, the present chapter focuses on the literature on depressed mothers who are characterized by an emotional depressive style such as those suffering from postpartum depression.

Moreover, as stated by Caroll Izard (1991), a depressed mood cannot be described in terms of sadness alone. It is a complex combination of different negative affects: *"The fundamental emotions involved in the phenomenology of depression are sadness – the key emotion – and anger, disgust, and contempt, fear, guilt, and shyness [...] There are other factors that are frequently present – decreased sexuality, decreased physical well-being and increased fatigue."* (Izard, 1991, p. 218). There is now ample evidence that all these negative moods and negative emotions affect both physical and mental functioning in depressed mothers via a series of cortical, somatic and autonomic responses. They therefore disrupt many social and cognitive behaviors (e.g. Beukeboom & Semin, 2006; Gil & Droit-Volet, 2009). Among these behaviors, those involved in initial child care and education in general have been identified. Depressed mothers have indeed been found to be characterized by insensitivity, unresponsiveness, negativity, and disengagement (e.g. Cohn et al., 1986; Field, 1984, 1986). They exhibit either no affect or negative affects. Consequently, they exhibit a mechanical form of childcare as if they were simply rigidly adhering to the rules of infant care. Many studies have further examined and coded mother-infant interactions in terms of attentiveness and shared affective states. Figure 3 shows the results found in Field's study (Field et al., 1990). The results of this study indicate that mother-infant dyads are characterized by a higher level of angry behavior and disengagement, and fewer periods of play when the mother is depressed rather than non-depressed. Moreover, Field also reported that depressed mothers spend less time engaged in shared behavior states (40%) than their non-depressed counterparts (54%).

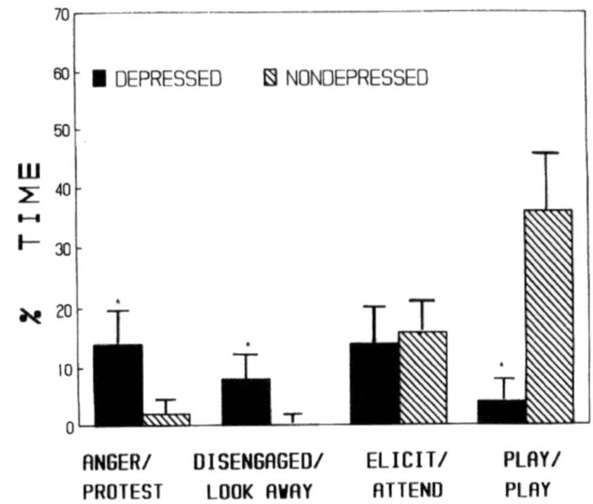


Fig. 3. Percentage of time that mothers and their infants shared behavior states, in 48 depressed mother-infant pairs and 48 nondepressed mother-infant pairs. Source: Field, Healy, Goldstein and Guthertz (1990).

Using self-report questionnaires, Righetti-Veltema and her colleagues (2002) showed that these depressed mothers are, in some respects, aware of their difficulties. They reported experiencing more difficulty in performing everyday activities with their 3-months-old infants. They also evaluated their behavior as more negative, and found their infants more demanding than non-depressed mothers. In line with this self-evaluation reported by depressed mothers, Lovejoy, Graczyk, O'Hare and Neuman's (2000) quantitative review of 46 observational studies conducted both in laboratory and home settings identified three types of maternal depression-related behaviors which have been categorized as disturbed: negative/coercive behaviors, positive behaviors and disengagement. Focusing more on emotional expressiveness, Martinez et al. (1996) videotaped infant-mother interactions and found that depressed mothers were indeed less expressive than non-depressed mothers, both when interacting with their own children and with the children of non-depressed mothers. Moreover, a number of studies have shown that depressed mothers produce fewer positive facial expressions and more neutral and negative facial expressions than non-depressed mothers (e.g. Cohn et al., 1986; Dawson et al., 2003; Field, 1992). Nevertheless, it is important to note that not all mothers with a similar level of depressive symptoms interact with their babies in the same way. Various studies have documented two distinct styles among depressed mothers which are referred to as "withdrawn" and "intrusive" (Cohn et al., 1990; Field et al., 1996; Field et al., 1990; Jones et al., 1997; Tronick, 1989). These two disruptive interactive styles are assumed to correspond to either understimulating or overstimulating behaviors. More precisely, the withdrawn mothers display fewer facial expressions. They are, in general, disengaged and unresponsive. In contrast, intrusive mothers are engaged but in a negative way. Although they exhibit emotional expressions, these are mostly negative, for example angry or irritated. They also commonly produce negative behaviors such as rough handling. However, as Field et al. (2006) add, 21% of depressed mothers do not correspond to either of these profiles. Nonetheless, whatever the interactive style, there is ample evidence that depressed mothers manifest maladaptive behaviors toward their babies.

## 4. The consequences of atypical mother-child interactions for infants' socio-emotional development

As reported above, mothers suffering from depression find it difficult to respond to their babies' needs and to communicate with them. The scientific literature suggests that this initial dysfunctioning of mother-baby relationships affects children's development by impairing babies' psychomotor and socio-emotional development. Embodiment theories suggest that, if they are to develop their own socio-emotional skills, children need to perform embodied simulations of emotions expressed by others, and in particular those expressed by the mother who is the focal point of this first social relationship (Niedenthal et al., submitted). Within this framework, the large number of negative emotional cues perceived by the babies of depressed mothers, both in terms of facial expression and comprehension, seems to cause such children to exhibit "atypical" emotional behavior and competences from the first months (Murray et al., 1999). Below, we report the various studies that can help explain or reveal how and why the behavior of depressed mothers can have consequences for their babies and their socio-emotional development.

There is ample evidence that the majority of mothers primarily display positive emotions when interacting with their infants. For example, in a well-designed experiment, Malatesta and Haviland (1982) reported that, during a six-minute period of interaction, mothers displayed 100 times more happiness than anger, and 40 times more anger than sadness. This positive attitude toward infants is assumed to contribute to attachment. As Bowlby (1951) has argued, attachment is *"essential for mental health in that an infant or young child should experience a warm, intimate and continuous relationship with (his or her) mother in which both find satisfaction and enjoyment"*. Attachment thus plays a critical role in how infants develop at the emotional level and how they cope with their social environment. Mary Ainsworth et al. (1978) has operationalized this concept attachment in a "strange situation paradigm" in which the infant is alternately in the presence of his or her mother or a stranger. Ainsworth identified different kinds of behavioral patterns in babies as a function of the quality of attachment, namely secure or insecure. In the strange situation, *secure attachment* causes the child to protest when his or mother leaves but to welcome her warmly again when she returns. The mother remains the reference point throughout the situation and the child continuously seeks her contact and proximity. In such cases, the mother is perfectly capable of responding adequately to her child's needs. In contrast, in the case of insecure attachment, Ainsworth distinguishes between three different styles (avoidance, ambivalent/resistant, and disorganized). However, all of these different insecure attachment styles are associated with a similar disruption in the child's behavior in the strange situation, i.e. the child is disturbed when the mother returns but not when she leaves. This specific type of reaction on the part of children is thought to result from their mothers' unresponsiveness or negative responses during everyday life. For our purposes here, it should be noted that maternal depression has been repeatedly linked to insecure parent-child attachments (Murray, 1992; Radke-Yarrow et al., 1985). In addition, longitudinal studies have revealed that postnatal depression has a harmful effect on infants during the first months of life and that these persists at school age. This phenomenon has been explained primarily in terms of the insecure nature of attachment between the infant and the depressed mother during the first few months following birth. Within this perspective, infants aged 18 months should be more likely to exhibit an insecure style of attachment if their mothers were depressed when their children were aged 2 months (Murray, 1992). Moreover, Murray and collaborators (1999) examined whether the behavior of 5-year-olds at home with their mothers or at school with their peers is indeed predicted by the mother's postnatal depression and the insecure attachment observed at 18 months. Their analyses of mediation confirmed that children's attitudes at the age of 5 years are predicted by the mother's depression and mediated by the initial style of attachment (Murray et al., 1999).

With reference to the regulation of the infant-adult dyad, a considerable body of literature has examined how the two partners develop what theorists call attunement or synchrony. These two terms refer to the fact that, during their interactions, mothers and infants establish coordinated behaviors that help bring about a behavioral and physiological harmony based on contingency. Within this framework, researchers have examined infants' responses to the atypical maternal behavioral characteristics of depressed mothers, i.e. negativity, unresponsiveness. One commonly employed paradigm is the non-contingent maternal behavior paradigm (Nadel et al., 1999). This procedure consists of three phases: (1) infant-mother interactions are initially videotaped during a free play period; (2) the mother's videotaped behavior is played back to the infant with the result that the infant-mother behavior is now non-contingent; and, finally, (3) a return to the free play situation, i.e. to natural contingent interactions. Similarly, Tronick et al. (1978) used the still-face paradigm which employs the same three phases, except that in the second phase, the recorded mother suddenly displays a neutral, motionless face. Using these two paradigms, many studies have shown that in the second phase, infants generally exhibit negative emotions, produce stressful behaviors and cry because they perceive a violation of harmonious interactions. They thus react negatively to this breakdown in natural communication (Muir et al., 2005; Tronick, 2005). In contrast, the infants of depressed mothers have been found to exhibit atypical behaviors and to produce fewer negative reactions in the disrupt phase. This is probably due to the fact that they are familiar with atypical rhythms of communication, i.e. those associated with their depressed mothers. They have grown accustomed to a lack of responsiveness and to passivity on the part of their depressed mother and to a low level of exposure to positive emotions (e.g. Field et al., 2005; Field et al., 2007; Pelaez-Nogueras et al., 1996).

As far as emotional behavior *per se* in children of depressed mothers is concerned, Reissland and Shepherd (2006) have shown that the infants of depressed mothers are also unresponsiveness to various situations in which emotions are elicited. These authors designed a play situation involving mothers and their children in the presence of a toy assumed to produce surprise: a Jack-in-the-box. Their results showed that the infants of mothers who reported a depressed mood were unreactive and displayed fewer emotional facial expressions than those of non-depressed mothers. The atypical behavior of infants therefore "mirrors" their mothers' unresponsiveness. Indeed, several studies have reported dysfunctions in the regulation of affects in the babies of depressed mothers, thus suggesting that they mirror the mother's mood. The babies of depressed mothers are indeed reported to be particularly likely to produce negative expressions, irritability and inconsolable screaming (Britton, 2011; Field, 1994; Hanington et al., 2010; Zuckerman et al., 1990).

Recent neuroscientific studies have provided arguments in support of the behavioral measures that indicate the presence of emotion disturbances in the babies of depressed mothers. More precisely, a right-frontal asymmetry in EEG activation has been observed in depressive individuals and more generally in states characterized by high levels of negative affects. There is now growing evidence that this specific pattern of brain activation is also found in the babies of depressed mothers. Furthermore, this specific activation of the right-frontal cortex is observed as of the very first months of life (i.e. 1 month) and continues to be present up to preschool age, (i.e. 3-years old) (Diego et al., 2004; Jones et al., 2000; Jones et al., 1997ab; Jones et al., 2009). Figure 4 illustrates the results obtained by Diego et al. These clearly show a greater right-frontal EEG activation in the infants of depressed mothers than in those of non-depressed mother when they are presented with different emotional expressions. In addition, as reported above, this specific pattern of brain activity in the infants of depressed mothers has been observed not only in response to their mothers' faces but also in response to the faces of unknown women, and is thus consistent with a generalization process. In other words, the general processing of emotional cues, in this case facial expressions, seems to be disrupted in these children.

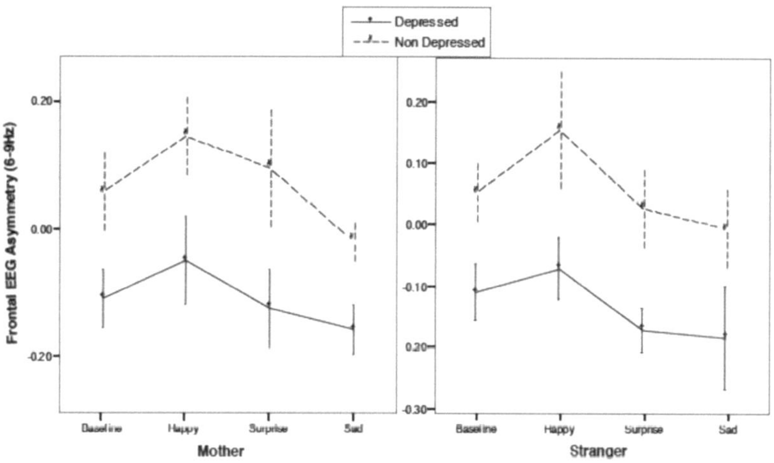


Fig. 4. Mean frontal EEG asymmetry (i.e. 6-9 Hz) of infants of depressed or non-depressed mothers in response to baseline, happy, surprised, sad expressions modeled by their mother (left panel) or an unknown female (right panel); positive values reflect greater left frontal EEG activation, negative scores reflect relatively greater right frontal EEG activation. Source: Diego et al. (2004).

Using experimental procedures more specifically designed to examine babies' emotional recognition competences, numerous studies have confirmed deficits in the processing of emotional facial expressions in the babies of depressed mothers. Based on the finding that infants look longer at new than at familiar stimuli, researchers have used the habituation paradigm to study the ability of babies to discriminate different emotional expressions. In this paradigm, infants are habituated through the repeated presentation of an initial stimulus (e.g. neutral face). Following habituation, i.e. when the time they spend looking at this initial stimulus has significantly decreased, they are presented with a second, new stimulus (e.g. happy face). If they look for significantly longer at the new stimulus, thus exhibiting what is referred to as a "novelty preference", this means that they discriminate between the two types of expression. The literature based on this and related paradigms provides considerable evidence that 4/5-month-old infants are able to discriminate a wide range of emotional expressions (e.g. Bornstein & Arteberry, 2003; Montague & Walker-Andrews, 2001; Serrano et al., 1992). Moreover, the few studies that have been conducted among the babies of depressed mothers have revealed that their ability to discriminate emotional expressions is impaired or atypical (e.g. de Haan et al., 2004; Lundy et al., 1997; Striano et al., 2002). For example, the results obtained by Bornstein et al. (2011) and presented in Figure 5, showed that whereas 5 month-old infants of non-depressed mothers are able to discriminate between happy and neutral faces, this ability is impaired in the infants of depressed mothers.

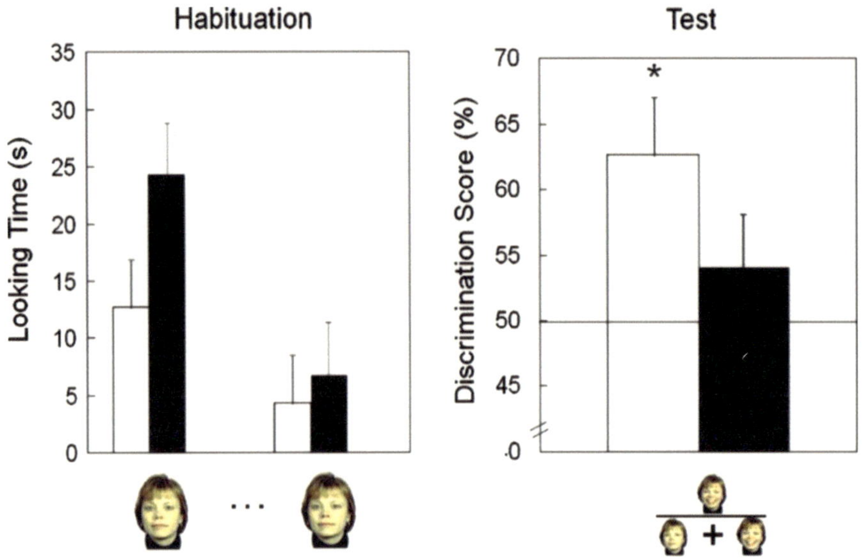


Fig. 5. Habituation (left panel) and novelty responsiveness (right panel) in infants of non-depressed (white bars) and depressed (black bars) mothers. Source: Bornstein et al. (2011).

However, even though there is a general consensus that the infants of depressed mothers perform worse in emotional tasks than the infants of non-depressed mothers, it should be noted that the results and the interpretations of them remain contradictory. For example, using a habituation paradigm, Striano et al. (2002) showed that the 6-month-old infants of depressed mothers preferred to look at happy faces. Using a matching task, Lundy et al. (1997) also showed that, unlike the 10-month-old babies of non-depressed mothers, those of depressed mothers performed less well on happy than on sad faces and preferred to look at the latter rather than the former. These different results lead to two contrasting interpretations. On the one hand, it can be claimed that the children of depressed mothers prefer smiling faces because their mothers do not often display this emotion (i.e. the salience hypothesis). On the other, it can be argued that these infants display a preference for sad expressions because they directly correspond to the usual mode of communication observed in depressed mothers (i.e. the exposure hypothesis). Further investigations will therefore be required if we are to successfully validate one or other of these hypotheses. However, whatever the explanation, the socio-emotional environment of the children of depressed mothers is different than that of other children and consequently results in different social behaviors and different patterns of socio-emotional development. In addition, the pathology of depressed mothers may also mean that they have to cope with difficulties in responding appropriately to and understanding their infants' needs. If this line of argument is correct then not only would depressed mother send out negative emotional cues to their children, but they would also have difficulty understanding the emotions expressed by them. Having now presented the results relating to children and their socio-emotional abilities, we will now focus more on the results relating to mothers.

## 5. Emotional processing in depressed mothers

The literature reporting studies of depressed individuals shows that they perform poorly when asked to evaluate emotional faces (George et al., 1998; Gur et al., 1992; Leppänen et al., 2004; Mendlewicz et al., 2005; Rubinow & Post, 1992; Suslow et al., 2001). This poorer performance is generally explained in terms of a bias in the processing of emotional cues. One initial type of bias takes the form of an attention-bias effect, with a depressed mood producing a selective attention-bias toward negative or mood-congruent incoming stimuli (e.g. sad faces). Negative cues are therefore processed faster than positive cues (Gotlib et al., 2004; Suslow et al., 2001). In addition, depressed individuals find it difficult to shift their attentional focus away from the negative cues. A second type of bias takes the form of the "mood congruence effect" and suggests that we see the world though the prism of our own mood (Niedenthal et al., 2000). While someone in love sees life through rose-tinted spectacles, the spectacles worn by depressed individuals are grey. This mood congruence effect explains why neutral faces are evaluated as negative, and negative faces as more negative by depressed compared to non-depressed individuals (Demenescu et al. 2010; Gollan et al., 2008; Gur et al., 1992). Finally, people with depression generally achieve poorer performances when asked to evaluate emotional faces (George et al., 1998; Gur et al., 1992; Leppänen et al., 2004; Mendlewicz et al., 2005; Rubinow & Post, 1992; Suslow et al., 2001).

One recent line of research to emerge from this literature has focused on mothers' emotional processing of their environments. The assumption is that if mothers with depression experience difficulties or exhibit atypical behavior when processing their babies' faces, this may explain why they experience problems in interacting with them. Reasoning within this framework, Stein et al. (2009) suggested that insensitivity or maladaptive adjustment between depressed mothers and their children would effectively be due to an attention-bias. More precisely, these authors describe mothers as being "preoccupied", a state that consumes all their attentional resources. They define preoccupation as *"a state of narrowed or self-focused attention in which one's mind is dominated by recurrent negative intrusive thoughts that are difficult to control, difficult to dismiss and recur even if dismissed"* (Stein et al., 2009, p.12). This working memory load explains distortions in the processing of information such as the mood congruence effect which is thought to lead to the preferential processing of congruent stimuli. It also explains why depressed mothers are less available for their children than non-depressed mothers. However, some caution must be exercised when attempting to generalize from general depression to postpartum depression because the processing of information in depressed mothers may exhibit specific characteristics related to their maternal status and their close relationships with their babies.

Surprisingly, as far as postnatal depression *per se* and its impact on emotional face processing are concerned, only four experimental studies have been published in recent years. In 2011, Flanagan and his colleagues examined potential impairments in the perception of emotional faces by women with postpartum depression, non-postpartum depression and female control subjects. These authors presented their participants with emotional facial expressions of adults displaying anger, fear, happiness and disgust. They showed that depressed women - of both postpartum and non-postpartum type - performed less well than the controls. Furthermore, the results revealed a difference in impairment as a function of the type of depression, with the postpartum-depressed women achieving poorer performances in the processing of disgusted and fearful faces, and the women with a different type of depression performing less well when asked to process happy faces. This study is therefore valuable in that it reveals that, as reported in the literature on depression, postpartum depression involves the atypical processing of emotional faces. However, the question that needs to be addressed by developmental psychologists is whether this atypical processing is also observed in response to infants' faces. Two other studies have therefore attempted to examine this question by presenting valence-related infant faces (positive, muted positive, neutral, muted negative and negative) (Stein et al., 2010), and morphed discrete-emotional faces (happy *vs.* sad faces) (Arteche et al., 2011). The results of Stein's study involving faces of infants showed that the depressed mothers evaluated infant faces expressing a negative emotion more negatively than the female controls, but that this was only the case when the participants saw the faces for a long (2000 ms) rather than a short (100 ms) period of time. Moreover, these results also suggest that depression was the only factor explaining the atypical response to the emotional faces. Neither comorbid postnatal psychopathology nor anxiety had an impact. Conversely, the study conducted by Arteche et al. (2011) indicated that depressed mothers were less accurate than female controls in identifying the faces of happy infants, with the performance on sad faces being unrelated to the depressive mood. Finally, Gil and colleagues (2011) addressed a related question: is the impairment in the processing of faces in women with postpartum depression greater in response to infant than to adult faces. To do this, these authors asked mothers who had only recently given birth (i.e. on the third day after delivery) to perform an emotional facial expressions task involving both adult and baby faces, each expressing the emotion of anger, happiness, sadness and fear (see Figure 6). Unlike Stein's findings, their results revealed differences in the recognition of negative emotions when these were displayed by baby and adult faces. In line with the mood congruence hypothesis, the women with postpartum depression judged the neutral baby faces to be less neutral and sadder than the control subjects. In addition, anxiety, as measured by the State-Trait Anxiety Inventory (STAI), and which was found to be greater in the women with postpartum depression than in the controls, appears to play a critical role in the evaluation of emotions (Spielberger et al., 1983). As the level of anxiety increased, both the neutral and angry facial expressions were indeed judged to be more disgusted. However, this was the case for both the infant and the adult faces.

Consequently, depression during the early postpartum period distorts the way mothers interpret children's facial expressions. Recent neuroscientific studies have shown that this depression affects the interpretation not only of the visual signals produced by babies but also of their auditory signals, such as their cries. In a pioneering study, Lorberbaum and colleagues (1999) used magnetic resonance imaging to investigate activity in the mother's brain in response to hearing a baby cry or listening to a white noise for 30 s. This study has

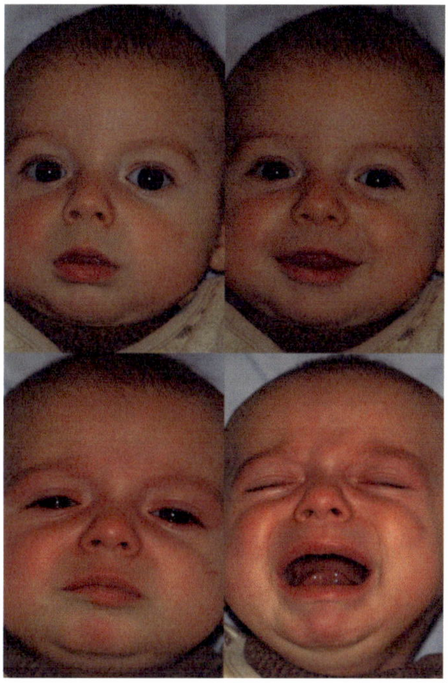

Fig. 6. Examples of babies' emotional facial expressions presented to mothers: neutrality, happiness, sadness, anger, in Gil et al.'s study (2011).

since been replicated by other studies which have used the crying of different babies, namely the mother's own child and that of another infant. All these studies have systematically shown that mothers' brains exhibit a higher level of activation than those of female controls when they hear their own baby crying (Lorberbaum et al., 2002; Purhonen et al., 2001). In addition, the activated brain regions are those related to alertness, empathy and/or the regulation of emotions. Unfortunately this new area of neuroscientific research has not as yet yielded any significant findings with regard to the postpartum depressive mood. Nonetheless, Swain and his team in 2008 have not directly address the question of postpartum depression, but a complementary one. In the same way as in conventional research, the authors scanned mothers some 2 to 4 weeks after giving birth when hearing babies crying (either their own or other babies), taking account of the mode of delivery. The mode of delivery is indeed considered as being a crucial factor contributing to the mother's mood. Delivery by cesarean section is thought to increase the risk of postpartum depression compared to vaginal delivery (Lobel & Deluca, 2007). The authors found that the brains of mothers who had given birth by means of cesarean section were less responsive to the crying of their own babies' cries than those of mothers who had experienced vaginal delivery. Only the insula was more activated in the mothers who had given birth by cesarean section. It is interesting to note that the literature on emotions reports that the insula is specifically involved in the processing of negative emotions, such as distress, pain or disgust (Adolphs et al., 2003; Craig et al., 2003; Wicker et al., 2003). This study therefore shows that mothers at risk of a depressive symptomatology are biologically less sensitive to their own babies' signals. However, the link between cesarean section and depression is still unclear (Carter et al., 2006), and the depression scores reported in this study are inversely related to the mode of delivery.

Whatever the case may be, the specific characteristics exhibited by mothers with postpartum depression in response to the visual and auditory emotional signals given by their babies has led psychologists to consider that the quality of the mother-infant relationship is impaired (for a review, see Swain, 2011). Researchers even speak about a particular parental pattern that can be observed in depressed mothers, in the same way as for the insecure style of attachment. Within this framework, Swain (2011) has, on the basis of studies conducted in humans and animals, proposed an integrative model of "the parental brain" that identifies the information processing operations and associated brain structures thought to govern parenting behaviors (see Figure 7). In this model, (A) the first step involves the sensory signals emitted by babies that are essential for parenting and which are then (B) detected by sensory cortices of the parent's brain. This first appraisal of infant stimuli is assumed, with enough motivation, to activate brain circuits (C) that are referred to as cortico-limbic modules. These modules refer to three kinds of cognitive activity and the associated brain structures: (I) the interaction between the reflexive caring functions, (II) high-level cognitive processes and (III) emotion-related mechanisms that produce a parental output behavior (D). In addition, due to feedback, the type of parental output behavior may modify the infant's behavior and the subsequent infant input stimuli, thus establishing a specific mother-child relationship. In the case of post-partum depression, we may suppose that mothers might find it difficult to accurately detect and process the input signals received from their babies due to their disturbed cognitive processes and underlying cortical structures. This might in turn lead to inappropriate output behaviors on the part of the mothers which might ultimately affect the input received from the infants. However, future research will be required in order to further investigate the question of the links between parental behavior and brain structures in mothers with postpartum depression and their evolution during different periods of child development.

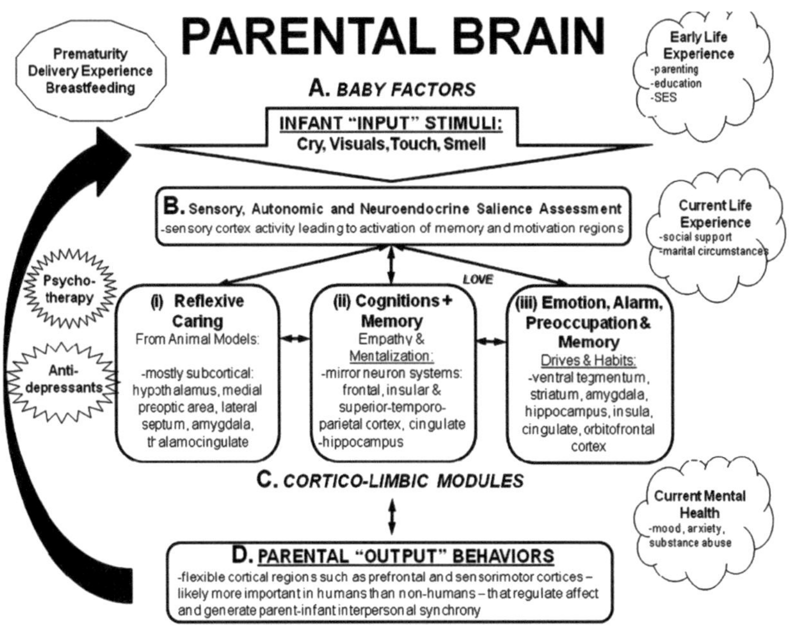


Fig. 7. The parental brain model: brain regions thought to be important for human parenting. Source: Swain (2011).

## 6. Conclusion

An examination of the ability and readiness of both mothers and infants to deal with emotional expressiveness in cases where the mother suffers from depression shows that, as of an early stage, depression affects the relationship between the two partners. Indeed, as we have reported, depressed mothers experience difficulties in their emotional communication with their children and exhibit atypical behavior, especially at the level of emotional facial expressions. For their part, the babies of such mothers exhibit impairments and dysregulations in their socio-emotional development in both the short and long term. However, few studies have examined the long-term effect of depressed mothers on children once they have acquired verbal language and found other persons of attachment. Indeed, many different factors may potentially compensate for the initial difficulties experienced by these babies. In addition, many questions remain unresolved, for example relating to the role of the father in the mother-child relationship when the mother is suffering from depression

To summarize, because the first few months following birth represents a sensitive and critical period for children's socio-emotional development, it is very important to be able to detect mothers who present a depressive symptomatology as early as possible so that both they and their children can be given the care required in order to counteract the emotional consequences of postpartum depression for both the mother and the child. The socio-emotional development of children and the various problems associated with depressive mothers therefore represent an important research domain which deserves further investigation.

## 7. Acknowledgements

This work was supported by a grant from the Agence Nationale de la recherche (ANR) "Emotion(s), cognition, comportement" from France

## 8. References

Adolphs, R., Tranel, D., & Damasio, A.R. (2003). Dissociable neural systems for recognizing emotions. *Brain Cognition, 52*, 61-69.

Ainsworth, M.D.S., Blehar, M.C., Waters, E., & Wall, S. (1978). *Patterns of attachment: A psychological study of the Strange Situation.* Hillsdale, NJ: Lawrence Erlbaum Associates.

American Psychiatry Association (APA) (1994). *Diagnostic and Statistical Manual of Mental Disorders,* 4th edition (DSM-IV), Washington, DC.

Arteche, A., Joormann, J., Harvey, A., Craske, M., Gotlib, I.H., Lehtonen, A., Counsell, N., & Stein, A. (2011). The effects of postnatal maternal depression and anxiety on the processing of infant faces. *Journal of Affective Disorders.*

Bandura, A. (1992). Social cognitive theory of social referencing. In S. Feinman (Ed.), *Social referencing and the social construction of reality in infancy* (pp. 175-208). New York: Plenum Press.

Batki, A., Baron-Cohen, S., Wheelwright, S., Connellan, J., & Ahluwalla, J. (2000). Is there an innate gaze module? Evidence from human neonates. *Infant Behavior and Development, 23*, 223-229.

Beck, C.T. (2002). Postpartum depression: a metasynthesis. *Qualitative Health Research, 12*, 453–472.

Beukeboom, C.J., & Semin, G.R. (2006). How mood turns on language. *Journal of Experimental Psychology, 42,* 553-566.
Bornstein, M.H., & Arteberry, M.E. (2003). Recognition, discrimination and categorization of smiling by 5-month-old infants. *Developmental Science, 6,* 585-599.
Bornstein, M.H., Arteberry, M.E., Mash, C., & Manian, N. (2011). Discrimination of facial expression by 5-month-old infants of nondepressed and clinically depressed mothers. *Infant Bahavior and Development, 34,* 100-106.
Bowlby, J. (1951). *Maternal Care and Mental Health. W.* H. O. Monographs, No. 2. London: H. M. Stationary Office; New York: Columbia University Press.
Bowlby, J. (1969). Attachment and loss: Vol. 1. *Attachment.* New York: Basic Books.
Britton, J.R. (2011). Infant temperament and maternal anxiety and depressed mood in the early postpartum period. *Women & Health, 51,* 55-71.
Camras, L.A., Malatesta, C., & Izard, C.E. (1991). The development of facial expressions in infancy. In S. Feldman & B. Rimé (Eds.), *Fundamentals of nonverbal behavior,* pp. 73-115. Cambridge: Cambridge University Press.
Carter, F.A., Frampton, C.M.A., & Mulder, R.T. (2006). Cesarean section and postpartum depression: a review of the evidence examining the link. *Psychosomatic Medicine, 68,* 321-330.
Chabrol, H., & Teissèdre, F. (2004). Relation between Edinburgh Postnatal Depression Scale scores at 2–3 days and 4–6 weeks postpartum. *Journal of Reproductive and Infant Psychology, 22,* 33–39.
Cohn, J.F., Campbell, S.B., Matias, R., & Hopkins, J. (1990). Face-to-face interactions of postpartum depressed and nondepressed mother-infant pairs at 2 months. *Developmental Psychology, 26,* 15-23.
Cohn, J.F., Matias, R., Tronick, E.Z., Connell, D., & Lyons-Ruth, K. (1986). Face-to-face interactions of depressed mothers and their infants. *New Directions for Child Development, 34,* 31-45.
Craig, A.D. (2003). Interoception: the sense of the physiological condition of the body. *Current Opinion in Neurobiology, 13,* 500-505.
Darwin, C. (1998). *The expression of the emotions in man and animals.* Oxford, England: Oxford University Press. (Original work published1872)
Dawson, G., Ashman, S., Pangiotides, H., Hessl, D., Self, J., Yamada, E., & Embry, L. (2003). Preschool outcomes of children of depressed mothers: Role of maternal bahavior, contextual risk, and children's brain activity. *Child Development, 74,* 1158-1175.
De Haan, M., Belsky, J., Reid, V., Volein, A., & Johnson, M.H. (2004). Maternal personality and infants' neural and visual responsivity to facial expressions of emotion. *Journal of Child Psychology and Psychiatry, 45,* 1209-1218.
Demenescu, L.R., Kortekaas, R., den Boer, J.A., & Aleman, A. (2010). Impaired attribution of emotion to facial expressions in anxiety and major depression. *PLoS ONE,* 5: e15058. doi:10.1371/journal.pone.0015058.
Diego, M.A., Field, T., Jones, N.A., Hernandez-Reif, M., Cullen, C., Schanberg, S., & Kuhn, C. (2004). EEG responses to mock facial expressions by infants of depressed mothers. *Infant Behavior and Development, 27,* 150-162.
Ekman, P. (1982). *Emotion in the human face.* New York: Pergamon Press.
Field, T. (1984). Early interactions between infants and their postpartum depressed mothers. *Infant Behavior and Development, 7,* 517-522.
Field, T. (1986). Models of reactive and chronic depression. In E. Tronick & T. Field (Eds.), *Maternal depression and infant disturbance* (pp. 47-60). San Francisco: Jossey-Bass.
Field, T. (1992). Infants of depressed mothers. *Development and Psychopathy, 4,* 49-66.

Field, T. (1994). The effects of mother's physical and emotional unavailability of emotion regulation. *Monographs of the Society for Research in Child Development, 59*, 208-227.
Field, T., Healy, B., Goldstein, S., & Guthertz, M. (1990). Behavior state matching in mother-infant interactions of nondepressed versus depressed mother-infant dyads. *Developmental Psychology, 26*, 7-14.
Field, T., Hernandez-Reif, M., Diego, M., Feijo, L., Gil, K., Sanders, C. (2007). Still-face separation effects on depressed mother-infant interactions. *Infant Mental Health Journal, 28*, 314-323.
Field, T., Lang, C., Martinez, A., Yando, R., Pickens, J., Bendell, D. (1996). Preschool follow-up of infants of dysphoric mothers. *Journal of Clinical Child Psychology, 25*, 272-279.
Field, T., Nadel, J., Hernadez-Reif, M., Diego, M., Vera, Y., Gil, K., Diego, M., & sanders, C. (2005). Depressed mothers' infants show less negative affect during non-contingent interactions. *Infant Behavior and Development, 28*, 426-430.
Flanagan, T.J., White, H., & Carter, B.G. (2010). Differential impairments in emotion face recognition in postpartum and nonpostpartum depressed woemn. *Journal of Affective Disorders, 128*, 314-318.
Frijda, N. H. (2007). *The laws of emotion*. Mawwah, NJ: Erlbaum.
Gil, S., & Droit-Volet, S. (2009). Time perception, depression and sadness. *Behavioural Processes, 80*, 169-176.
Gil, S., Teissèdre, F., Chambres, P., & Droit-Volet, S. (2011). The evaluation of emotional facial expressions in early postpartum depressive mood: A difference between adult and baby faces? *Psychiatry Research, 186, 281-286.*
Gollan, J.K., Pane, H., McCloskey, M., & Coccaro, E.F. (2008). Identifying differences in biased affectective information processing in major depression. *Psychiatry Research, 159*, 18-24.
Gonidakis, F., Rabavilas, A.D., Varsou, E., Kreatsas, G., & Christodoulou, G.N. (2008). A 6-month study of postpartum depression and related factors in Athens Greece. *Comprehensive Psychiatry, 49*, 275–282.
Goren, C.C., Sarty, M., & Wu, P.Y.K. (1975). Visual following and pattern discrimination of face-like stimuli by newborn infants. *Pediatrics, 56*, 544-549.
Gotlib, I.H., Krasnoperova, E., Yue, D.N., & Joormann, J. (2004). Attentional biases for negative interpersonal stimuli in clinical depression. *Journal of Abnormal Psychology, 113*, 127-135.
Gur, R.C., Erwin, R.J., Gur, R.E., Zwill, A.S., Heimberg, C., & Kraemer, H.C. (1992). Facial emotion discrimination: II. Behavioral findings in depression. *Psychiatry Research, 42*, 241-251.
Hanington, L., Ramchandani, P., & Stein, A. (2010). Parental depression and child temperament: Assessing child to parent effects in a longitudinal population study. *Infant Bahavior & Development, 33*, 88-95.
Hendrick, V., Altshuler, L., Strouse, T., & Grosser, S. (2000). Postpartum and nonpostpartum depression: Differences in presentation and response to pharmacologic treatment. *Depression and Anxiety, 11*, 66-72.
Hess, U. (2001). The communication of emotion. In A. Kaszniak (Ed.), *Emotions, Qualia, and Consciousness* (pp. 397-409). Singapore: World Scientific Publishing.
Izard, C. E. (1971). *The face of emotion*. New York: Appleton-Century-Crofts.
Izard, C.E. & Malatesta, C.Z. (1987). Perspectives on emotional development. I. Differential emotions theory of early emotional development. In J.D. Osofsky (Ed.), *Handbook of Infant Development* (2nd., pp. 494-554). New York: Wiley.

Johnson, M.H., Dziurawiec, S., Ellis, H., & Morton, J. (1991). Newborns' preferential tracking of face-like stimuli and its subsequent decline. *Cognition, 40*, 1-19.

Jones, N.A., Field, T., & Almeida, A. (2009). Right frontal EEG asymmetry and behavioural inhinbition in infants of depressed mothers. *Infant Behavior and Development, 32*, 298-304.

Jones, N.A., Field, T., & Davalos, M. (2000). Right frontal EEG asymmetry and lack of empathy in preschool children of depressed mothers. *Child Psychiatry and Human Development, 30*, 189-204.

Jones, N.A., Field, T., Davalos, M., & Pickens, J. (1997a). EEG stability in infants/children of depressed mothers. *Child Psychiatry and Human Development, 28*, 59-70.

Jones, N.A., Field, T., Fox, N.A., Lundy, B., & Davalos, M. (1997b). EEG activation in 1-month-old infants of depressed mothers. *Development and Psychopathology, 9*, 491-505.

Keltner, D. & Haidt, J. (2001). Social functions of emotions. In T. Mayne & G.A. Bonanno (Eds.), *Emotions: Current issues and future directions* (pp. 192–213). New York: Guilford Press.

Kugiumutzakis, G. (1998). Neonatal imitation in the intersubjective companion space. In B. Stein (Ed.), *Intersubjective communication and emotion in early ontogeny* (pp. 63-88). Cambridge University Press.

Leppänen, J.M., Milders, M., Bell, J.S., Terriere, E., & Hietanen, J.K. (2004). Depression biases the recognition of emotionally neutral faces. *Psychiatry Research, 128*, 123-133.

Leslie, A.M. (1987). Pretense and representation: The origins of "Theory of mind". *Psychological Review, 94*, 412-426.

Lobel, M., & Stein DeLuca, R. (2007). Psychosocial sequelae of cesarean delivery : Reviwe and analysis of their cuases and implications. *Social Sciences & Medecine, 64*, 2272-2284.

Loberbaum, J.P., Newman, J.D., Horwitz, A.R., Dubno, J.R., Lydiard, R.B., Hamner, M.B., Bohning, D.E., & George, M.S. (2002). A potential rôle for thalamocingulate cicuitry in human maternal behavior. *Society of Biological Psychiatry, 51*, 431-445.

Lovejoy, M.C., Graczyk, P.A., O'Hare, E., & Neuman, G. (2000). Maternal depression and parenting behavior: A meta-analytic review. *Clinical Psychology Review, 20*, 561-592.

Lundy, B., Field, T., Cigales, M., & Cuadra, A. (1997). Vocal and facial expression matching in infants of mothers with depressive symptoms. *Infant Medical Health Journal, 18*, 265-273.

Malatesta, C.Z., & Haviland, J.M. (1982). Learning display rules: The socialization of emotion expression in infancy. *Child Development, 53*, 991-1003.

Martinez, A., Malphurs, J., Field, T., Pickens, J., Yando, R., Bendell, D., Valle, C., & Messinger, D. (1996). Depressed mothers' and their infants' interactions with nondepressed partners. *Infant Mental Health Journal, 17*, 74-80.

Meltzoff, A.N., & Moore, M.K. (1977). Imitation of facial and manual gestures by human neonates. *Science, 198*, 75-78.

Mendlewicz, L., Linkowski, P., Bazelmans, C., & Phillippot, P. (2005). Decoding emotional facial expressions in depressed and anorexic patients. *Journal of Affective Disorders, 89*, 195-199.

Mondloch, C.J., Lewis, T.L., Budreau, D.R., Maurer, D., Dannemiller, J.L., Stephens, B.J., & Kleiner-Gathercoal, K.A. (1999). Face perception during early infancy. *Psychological Science, 10*, 419-422.

Montague, D.P.F., & Walker-Andrews, A.S. (2001). Peekaboo: a new look at infants' perception of emotion expressions. *Developmental Psychology, 37*, 826–838.

Muir, D., Lee, K., Hains, C., & Hains, S. (2005). Infant perception and production of emotions during face-to-face interactions with live and "virtual" adults. In J. Nadel & D. Muir (Eds.). *Emotional Development* (pp. 207-233). Oxford University Press.

Murray, L. (1992). The impact of postnatal depression on infant development. *Journal of Child Psychology and Psychiatry, 33,* 543-561.

Murray, L., Sinclair, D., Cooper, P., Ducournau, P., & Turner, P. (1999). The socioemotional development of 5-year-old children of postnatally depressed mothers. *Journal of Child Psychology and Psychiatry, 40,* 1259-1278.

Nadel, J., Carchon, I., Kervella, C., Marcelli, D., Réserbat-Plantey, D. (1999). Expectancies for social contingency in 2-month-olds. *Developmental Science, 2,* 164-173.

Niedenthal, P.M., Augustinova, M., Zinner, L., Rychlowska, M., Droit-Volet, S., & Brauer, M. (submitted). Emotional dummy? Pacifier users show compromised emotional competence.

Niedenthal, P.M., Halberstadt, J.B., Margolin, J., Innes-Ker, A.H. (2000). Emotional state and the detection of change in facial expression of emotion. *European Journal of Social Psychology, 30,* 211–222.

Papousek, H., & Papousek, M. (1978). Interdisciplinary parallels in studies of early human behaviour: From physical to cognitive needs, from attachment to dyadic education. *International Journal of Behavioural Development, 1,* 37-49.

Papousek, H., & Papousek, M. (1989). Forms and functions of vocal matching in interactions between mothers and their precanonical infants. *First Language, 9,* 137-158.

Pascalis, O., de Haan, M., & nelson, C.A. (2002). Is face processing species-specific during the first year of life? *Science, 296, 1321-1323.*

Pelaez-Nohueras, M., Field, T.M., Hossain, Z., & Pickens, J. (1996). Depressed mothers' touching increases infants' positive affect and attention in still-face interactions. *Child Development, 67,* 1780-1792.

Purhonen, M., Kllpelälnen-Lees, R., Valkonen-Korhonen, M., Karhu, J., Lehtonen, J. (2004). Cérébral processing of mother's voice compared to unfamiliar voice in 4-month-old infants. *International Journal of Psychophysiology, 52,* 257-266.

Radke-Yarrow, M., Cummings, E.M., Kuczynski, L., & Chapman, M. (1985). Patterns of attachment in two- and three-year-olds in noral families and families with parental dépression. *Child Development, 56,* 884-893.

Reissland, N., & Shepherd, J. (2006). The effect of maternal depressed mood on infant emotional reaction in a surprise-eliciting situation. *Infant mental health Journal, 27,* 173-187.

Reissland, N., Shepard, J., & Herrera, E. (2003). The pitch of maternal voice: a comparison of mothers suffering from depressed mood and non-depressed mothers reading books to their infants. *Journal of Child Psychology and Psychiatry, 43,* 1-7.

Righetti-Veltema, M., Conne-Perréard, E., Bousquet, A., & Manzano, J. (2002). Postpartum depression and mother-infant relationship at 3 months old. *Journal of Affective Disorders, 70,* 291-306.

Rosenstein, D., & Oster, H. (1988). Differential facial responses to four basic tastes in newborns. *Child Development, 59,* 1555-1568.

Rubinow, D.R., & Post, R.M. (1992). Impaired recognition of affect expression in depressed patients. *Biological Psychiatry, 31,* 947-953.

Russel, J.A., & Fernandez-Dols, J.M. (1997). *The psychology of facial expression.* Cambridge University Press.

Schoetzau, A., & Papousek, H. (1977). Maternal behavior in relation to the achievement of visual contact with newborn. *Zeitschrift für Entwicklungspsychologie und Pädagogische Psychologie, 9*, 231-239.
Serrano, J.M., Iglesias, J., & Loeches, A. (1992). Visual discrimination and recognition of facial expressions of anger, fear, and surprise in 4- to 6-month-old infants. *Developmental Psychobiology, 25*, 411–425.
Sit, D., Rothschild, A.J., & Wisner, K.L. (2006). A review of postpartum psychosis. *Journal of Women's Health, 15*, 352-368.
Spielberger, C.D., Gorsuch, R.L., Lusthene, R.E., 1983. *Manual for the State-Trait Anxiety Inventory*. Consulting Psychologist Press, Palo Alto.
Sroufe, L.A. (1996). *Emotional development: The organization of emotional life in the early years.* New York: Cambridge University Press.
Stein, A., Arteche, A., Lehtonen, A., Craske, M., Harvey, A., Counsell, N., & Murray, L. (2010). Interpretation of infant facial expression in the context of maternal postnatal depression. *Infant Behavior and Development, 33*, 273-278.
Stein, A., Lehtonen, A., Harvey, A.G., Nicol-Harper, R., & Craske, M. (2009). The influence of postnatal psychiatric disorder on child development: Is maternal preoccupation one of the key underlying processes? *Psychopathology, 42*, 11-21.
Striano, T., Brennan, P.A., & Vanman, E.J. (2002). Maternal depressive symptoms and 6-month-old infants' sensitivity to facial expressions. *Infancy, 3*, 115-126.
Suslow, T., Klauss, J., & Volker, A. (2001). Detection of facial expressions of émotions in dépression. *Perceptual and Motor Skills, 92*, 857-868.
Swain, J.E. (2011). The human parental brain: In vivo neuroimaging. *Progress in Neuro-Psychopharmacology & Biological Psychiatry, 35*, 1242-1254.
Swain, J.E., Tasgin, E., Mayes, L.C., Feldman, R., Constable, R.T., & Leckman, J.F. (2008). Maternal brain response to own baby-cry is affected by cesarean section delivery. *Journal of Child Psychology and Psychiatry, 49*, 1042-1052.
Trevarthen, C. (1979). Communication and cooperation in early infancy. A description of primary intersubjectivity. In M. Bullowa (Ed.), *Before speech: The beginning of human communication* (pp. 321-347). Cambridge: Cambridge University Press.
Trevarthen, C. (1998). The concept and foundations of infant intersubjectivity. In B. Stein (Ed.). *Intersubjective communication and emotion in early ontogeny* (pp. 15-46). Cambridge University Press.
Tronick, E. (2005). Why is connection with others so critical? The formation of dyadic states of cousciousness and the expansion of individuals' states of cousciousness: coherence governed selection and the co-creation of meaning out of messy meaning making. In J. Nadel & D. Muir (Eds.). *Emotional Development* (pp. 293-315). Oxford University Press.
Tronick, E., Als, H., Adamson, L., et al. (1978). The infants' response to entrapment between contradictory messages in face-to-face interactions. *Journal of the American Academy of Child Psychiatry, 17*, 1-13.
Tronick, E.Z. (1989). Emotions and emotional communication in infants. *American Psychologist, 44*, 112-119.
Wicker, B., Keysers, C., Plailly, J., Royet, J-P., Gallese, V., & Rizzolatti, G. (2003). Both of us disgusted in my insula: The common neural basis of seeing and feeling disgust. *Neuron, 40*, 655-664.
Zuckerman, B., Bauchner, H., Parker, S., & Cabral, H. (1990). Maternal depression symptoms during pregnancy, and newborn irritability. *Journal of Developmental and Behavioral Pediatrics, 11*, 190-194.

# 7

# Postpartum Depression and Maternity Blues in Immigrants

Fragiskos Gonidakis
*University of Athens, Medical School, 1st Psychiatric Department, Greece*

## 1. Introduction

Over the last decades the phenomenon of economic migration has increased significantly. The majority of immigrants are leaving their country mainly in order to improve their quality of life and work conditions.

A number of studies identify significantly elevated levels of psychological distress among immigrants than non-immigrant population (Mirsky, 2008, Taloyan et al, 2008). International migration has been characterized as a stressful life-event that causes an overburdening of the 'psychosomatic adjustment capacity', leading to higher emotional distress, diminished well-being and illness (Hull, 1979). The elevated psychological distress can affect directly the immigrants' everyday life leading to higher alcohol use, lower quality of life or even suicide ideation (Daher et al, 2011; Lindert et al, 2008). Most of the studies assessing immigrants' psychopathology have not focused on discrete psychiatric disorders but on general psychological distress, which includes anxiety, depressive feelings and somatisation. In a telephone survey conducted in Israel, 52% of adult immigrants reported depressive symptomatology compared to 38% of non-immigrants (Gross et al, 2001). Also, immigrant women were one-and-a-half times more likely than Israel born women to suffer from anxiety disorders (Mirsky et al, 2008). Furthermore, immigration as well as the adaptation process to the mainstream culture of the new country has been linked to mental disorders and especially depression (Gonidakis et al, 2011; Madianos et al, 2008, Sam, 2006a).

It has been well documented that immigration constitutes a stress factor that may influence the emotional status of women after delivery. Ozeki (2008) has reported that isolation, language and cultural barriers, and raising their children in a different cultural environment were the main stressors that Japanese mothers living in the United Kingdom were facing. Also Taniguchi and Baruffi (2009) have found that language barrier, distance from family and friends, different culture, and health-care attitude regarding childbirth were the stress factors reported by women from Japan who gave birth in Hawaii. A study conducted in Australia showed that immigrant women were more likely than Australian-born women to be breastfeeding at six months and were equally confident in caring for their baby and talking to health providers. No differences were found in anxiety or relationship problems with partners. However, compared with Australian-born women, immigrant mothers less proficient in English did have a higher prevalence of depression and were more likely to report seeking more practical and emotional support. They were more likely to have no 'time out' from baby care and to report feeling lonely and isolated (Bandyopadhyay, 2010).

Although there has been mounting research in mental disorders in the puerperium and especially postpartum depression, little focus has been placed on immigrant women (Fung and Dennis, 2010). This is a significant limitation given the continuous growth of the immigration movement and the changing demographics in North America and Europe. In Greece within two decades the percentage of the population that was born in another country has increased rapidly due to vast arrivals of immigrants from a large number of geographical areas such as the Balkans (Albania and Bulgaria), Eastern Europe (Poland, former USSR countries), Western and Eastern Africa (Nigeria and Ethiopia), and Western and Central Asia (Iraq, Afghanistan, Pakistan and Bangladesh). Most of these people have decided to immigrate for political, financial, and/or personal reasons, such as domestic violence or divorce. It is estimated that about 10% of the inhabitants of Athens are first generation immigrants. Furthermore, an unknown number of immigrants remain in Greece for only a short time, as their final destination is Central Europe or North America (Gonidakis et al, 2011).

## 2. Postpartum depression and immigration

Postpartum depression is one of the most common complications of childbearing. Most studies on postpartum depression have been conducted in developed countries and have reported a prevalence rate between 10-15% (Mann et al, 2010). Even though it has been suggested that postpartum depression might be more frequent in urban westernized societies, recent studies in non-western countries showed that postpartum depression has similar prevalence rates in different societies around the globe (Halbreich and Karkun, 2006). An international study that explored levels of postpartum depression in nine countries representing five continents showed that European and Australian women had the lowest levels, US women had intermediate and women from Asia and South America had the highest level of depressive symptoms (Affonso et al, 2000).

### 2.1 Prevalence rate of postpartum depression among immigrants

A growing body of research suggests that immigrant women may have higher rates of postpartum depression (Fung and Dennis, 2010). Steward et al (2008) have reported that postpartum depression occurred more often in immigrant, refugee and asylum seeking women that in native Canadian women. In a recent study conducted also in Canada Miszkurka et al (2010) found that immigrant women had a higher prevalence of depressive symptomatology independently of time since immigration. Mechakra-Tahiri et al (2007) have reported that in a study among immigrant women in Canada the prevalence of high depressive symptoms was larger among immigrants from minority groups than among immigrants from majority groups and Canadian-born mothers. Similar results have also been reported by Zelkowitz et al (2008).

However, there are studies in the literature that found lower frequency or no difference in the rates of postpartum depression among immigrant and native populations. Bjerke et al (2008) reported lower rates of postpartum depression in Pakistani women living in Norway.

The authors suggest that this result could be attributed to cultural differences in the perception of depressive symptomatology as mental illness, the presence of family members during the interview and the use of measurements in Norwegian rather than 'Urdu', the official Pakistani language. Davila et al (2009) found lower rates of postpartum depression in foreign-born Hispanic mothers living in USA when they were compared to US-born mothers. Finally, Kuo et al (2004) found that postpartum depression prevalence was not associated with the immigration status in a sample of Hispanic mothers living in USA.

The contradictory results from these studies highlight the complex interplay of social and cultural factors that may affect the risk of postpartum depression among immigrant women (Bhugra, 2003; Fung and Dennis, 2010).

### 2.2 Risk factors for postpartum depression among immigrant women

A number of reviews and meta-analyses suggest a multifactorial etiology for postpartum depression. The most common predictive factors are: previous history of depression, manifestation of maternity blues the first days after delivery and poor social and marital support (Beck, 2001, Robertson et al, 2004).

Similar factors have been related to the development of postpartum depression in immigrant mothers. Specifically, the relation of social support and the development of postpartum depression has been extensively investigated in immigrant populations. Stuchbery et al (1998) have conducted a study on social support and postpartum depression in a sample of Vietnamese, Arabic and Anglo-Celtic mothers living in Australia. The authors found that for Vietnamese mothers low postnatal mood was associated with poor quality of the relationship with the partner and a perceived need for more practical help from him. For Arabic women low postnatal mood was associated with perceived need for more emotional support from partners while for Anglo-Celtic women the need for emotional support was directed both to the partner and the woman's mother. Steward et al (2008) have reported that immigrant women with less prenatal support were more likely to develop depressive symptomatology after delivery. The authors suggest that lower social support could be the factor that increases the risk for postpartum depression in newcomers.

Prenatal depressive and somatic symptoms as well as marital quality were the best predictors of postpartum depressive symptomatology in immigrant women living in Canada (Zelkowitz et al, 2008). Miszkurka et al (2010) found that the region of origin was a strong predictor of depressive symptomatology: women from the Caribbean, South Asia, Maghreb, Sub-Saharan Africa and Latin America had the highest prevalence of depressive symptomatology compared to Canadian-born women. The higher depression odds in immigrant women were attenuated after adjustment for lack of social support and financial difficulties. Time trends of depressive symptoms varied across origins. In relation to length of stay, depressive symptoms increased (European, Southeast Asian), decreased (Maghrebian, Sub-Saharan African, Middle Eastern, East Asian) or fluctuated (Latin American, Caribbean). Furthermore, self-reported health, health beliefs, access to health care and adaptation to a new environment were fours key themes reported by Asian immigrant women in Taiwan who had developed postpartum depression (Huang and Mathers, 2008).

Finally it should be noted that many immigrant women have experienced extremely traumatizing events prior to immigration as well as stressful conditions during and after immigration. Some of these conditions are: lack of legal residence in the host country, unemployment, poor housing conditions and lack of autonomy. A qualitative study conducted among Asian mothers living in Canada showed that the migration experience as well as post-immigration stress was related to depressive symptomatology (Morrow et al, 2008). It is interesting that some of the women that were interviewed attributed the distress that they were experiencing to inadequate support from their husbands. In their home countries these women would first turn to their mothers and female relatives for support. After immigration the husband was usually the only person they could ask for help. But the husbands seemed to be ill-prepared for this change of their traditional role and in many cases they were unable to fulfill their wives' expectations (Morrow et al, 2008).

### 2.2.1 Acculturation and postpartum depression

A recurrent issue in studies on immigration and mental health is the role of culture as a health risk or protective factor, particularly the phenomenon of acculturation (Berry, 2006; Bhugra, 2004a, 2004b). In 2004, The International Organization for Migration defined acculturation as "the progressive adoption of elements of a foreign culture, ideas, words, values, norms, behaviors, institutions by persons, groups or classes of a given culture" (Sam, 2006a).

One fundamental issue in acculturation research is dimensionality. Two major models have been introduced in the literature (Sam, 2006a). The unidimensional model proposes that when an immigrant adopts elements of a mainstream culture, he/she moves away from his/hers own heritage culture (LaFromboise et al, 1993). In this model, acculturation and assimilation processes are viewed as similar (Bhugra, 2004a). The bidimensional model assumes that it is possible for an immigrant to acquire elements of the mainstream culture without losing his/her original culture (Berry, 1980). The bidimensional model separates heritage and mainstream acculturation as two processes that coexist in two different dimensions (Sam, 2006a).

Regardless of the model used to study and comprehend acculturation, a considerable amount of stress can arise as a result of immigrants' continuous and sometimes unsuccessful effort at social integration and acceptance by the mainstream culture (Berry, 2006). This effort includes learning the language and lifestyle of the mainstream culture, struggling to come to terms with homesickness and adaptation to the new country, overcoming financial and professional difficulties, or trying to function within a "new meaning" system. Furthermore, it is well established in the literature that chronic stress, such as acculturative stress, is linked with the manifestation of mental disorders, especially depression (Bale, 2006).

Previous studies have demonstrated an ambiguous relationship between acculturation and mental health, especially depressive mood (Sam, 2006b). The interplay between acculturation stress and postpartum depression has not been investigated extensively. In the literature there is only a small number of studies reporting contradictory results. Davila et al (2009) showed that higher acculturation in Latino mothers living in USA was associated with higher rates of postpartum depression. Abbot and Williams (2006), utilizing the bidemensional model of acculturation, showed that marginalized (low orientation to both host and heritage culture) Pacific Island women living in Australia had a significant higher risk of developing postpartum depression. Contrary to these results a study conducted in Hmong mothers living in the USA (Foss, 2001) and a study conducted in a population of immigrant mothers living in Canada (Zelkowitz et al, 2008) reported higher rates of postpartum depression in less acculturated mothers. It is interesting that a number of studies did not find any consistent relationship between acculturation and postpartum depression (Beck et al, 2005; Kuo et al, 2004).

The interpretation of these results needs to consider the complex nature of acculturation, the lack of widely accepted definition and measurements as well as the discrepancies among cultures and countries that may inhibit the generalizability of each study's results.

### 2.2.2 Postpartum depression and traditional rituals in immigrants

Traditional rituals concerning the puerperium exist in most cultures. Common practices include support for the mother, restricted activity, specific dietary and hygiene prescriptions that last about a month to forty days (Fung and Dennis, 2010, Grigoriadis et al, 2009). An example of traditional ritual is the japanese 'Satogaeri bunben'. 'Satogaeri' means returning to the original family town or house and 'bunben' means delivery. What actually happens is that the new mother after delivery returns for a period of 40 days to her mother's home so that she can be helped and cared by the older and more experienced woman. 'Satogaeri bunben' has not been found to lower the incidence of postpartum depression (Yoshida et al, 2001). A recent review on traditional postpartum rituals concluded that "there is some evidence that postpartum rituals dictating appropriate and wanted social support may be of some protective value, depending on numerous contextual factors" (Grigoriadis et al, 2009).

## 2.3 Barriers to research and identification of postpartum depression in immigrant populations

The research and identification of postpartum depression in immigrant populations is challenged by a number of factors:

1. The results from each study are difficult to be generalized. The factors that influence the development of postpartum depression in Mexican American women are not necessarily the same as the ones that have an impact on Albanian women living in Greece.
2. The use of scales to measure postpartum depression. There are three concerns regarding the issue of using translated instruments in transcultural studies (Nguyen et al., 2007). Specifically: (a) the instrument may fail to capture the conceptualization of postpartum depression in different cultural groups, (b) the instrument may include items that are irrelevant to the expression of postpartum depression in other cultural groups than the one for which it was designed, (c) factors such as social stigmatization, ethnicity, gender and age of the interviewer, and the setting of the interview may influence the way people respond.
3. Finally, a third limitation is the language barrier (Bhui and Bhugra, 2001). This is not only related to the level of knowledge of the host country's language, but also to semantic differences in the usage of the same words by people coming from different linguistic and cultural backgrounds.

## 3. The transcultural aspect of maternity blues

Maternity blues is a mild and transient phenomenon characterized mainly by feeling tearful, tired, anxious, forgetful, muddled, overemotional, changeable in mood, and low spirited, that occurs during the first days of puerperium (Gonidakis et al, 2007). Reports of the phenomenon exist since the late 19th century (Savage, 1875). In the early 50's, Moloney (1952) described a mild depressive reaction after delivery characterized by bursts of tears, fatigue and difficulty in thinking, which he named "third day depression" while in the 70's Pitt (1973) introduced the term "Maternity Blues". Although benign in nature maternity blues has been linked with the occurrence of postpartum depression, a mood disorder with substantial influence on the mother's welfare and the child's rearing (Darcy et al, 2011; Gonidakis et al, 2008).

Despite the large number of studies on mood disorders after delivery there is still no standard definition of maternity blues. The lack of diagnostic criteria, as well as the differences in the research methodology, are two of the main reasons for the wide range of prevalence rates that has been reported in various studies. Thus, the prevalence of maternity blues has been reported as high as 83% in a study from Tanzania (Harris, 1981) and as low as 8% in a study from Japan (Tsukashaki et al, 1991). Most of the authors agree that the prevalence of maternity blues varies between 40-60% (Hay and Levy, 2003; Nagata et al, 2000).

The fact that a number of studies reporting low prevalence of maternity blues are coming from Japan (Murata et al, 1998; Tsukashaki et al, 1991; Yoshida et al, 1997) has also raised the issue of cultural differences and especially the influence of culture in family support during puerperium. Nagata et al (2000) explored the effect of traditional support (satogaeri bunben) that Japanese women receive after delivery but found no correlation with the occurrence of maternity blues.

Although there are authors that have suggested that maternity blues is a cultural-bound syndrome that is observed mainly in western-type cultures where the traditional supportive rituals regarding the period of puerperium have subsided (Ugarizza, 1992), there has not been any conclusive evidence yet that the occurrence of maternity blues is related to socio-cultural factors (Kumar, 1994).

So far a number of psychosocial parameters have been tested in order to establish the risk factors of maternity blues. Most of the studies did not find any relation between the manifestation of the phenomenon and sociodemographic factors such as age, education, occupation and marital status (Nagata et al, 2000; O'Hara et al, 1991). Unwanted pregnancy, parity, caesarean section, breastfeeding and family support have also been tested but with contradictory results (Hensaw et al, 2003; Gonidakis et al, 2007). Negative emotions such as anxiety, fear of giving birth, and depression as well as stressful life events during pregnancy have been related to maternity blues (Bergant et al, 1998; Gonidakis et al, 2007; O'Hara et al, 1991; Pop et al, 1995).

## 4. Maternity blues and postpartum depression in a sample of Albanian women living in Athens, Greece

The present study, which was part of a larger study on maternity blues and postpartum depression in Greece (Gonidakis et al, 2007, 2008), attempts to investigate primarily maternity blues and postpartum depression in first generation immigrant mothers compared to a sample of native Greek women and secondly clinical and sociodemographic factors that are related with the occurrence of maternity blues and postpartum depression in immigrants. According to the literature review and the author's clinical experience acquired by treating immigrants, more immigrant than Greek women were expected to experience depressive symptomatology. Since, according to the author's knowledge, there are no other studies in the literature, that have dealt with the issue of maternity blues in immigrant mothers, the study had an exploratory nature and there was no hypothesis formulated prior to the investigation.

### 4.1 Methodology

The present cross-sectional study consists of two arms. The first concerns the prevalence of maternity blues during the first three days of puerperium and postpartum depression during the first three months after delivery as well as the factors related with the manifestation of these two mood disorders of the puerperium. The second arm concerns the comparison between two ethnic groups, an immigrant and a native Greek. The immigrant group consisted of women coming from Albania. the reasons behind this choice were two. The first was that Albanian immigrants is the largest immigrant group in Greece and the second is that Albanians and Greeks are two nations residing in the Balkan area in great cultural proximity, sharing many common customs and rituals concerning the period of pregnancy and puerperium.

#### 4.1.1 Participants

The study was conducted at the 1st Obstetrics and Gynecology Department of University of Athens, Medical School. The first 100 immigrant women, who consecutively gave birth in the department, were approached and examined the first day after delivery.

The inclusion criteria were adequate knowledge of the Greek language (to be able to speak and read in Greek), birth of a healthy child (Apgas score of 9-10), absence of personal history of psychotic disorder, use of psychoactive substances and chronic somatic disease. Also women that were suffering from depression at the time of the first examination (score higher than 20 in the Montgomery-Asberg Depression Rating Scale (Montgomery and Asberg, 1979) were excluded from the study. The above was decided in order to avoid misdiagnosing antenatal depression as postpartum depression or maternity blues.

Each immigrant woman that was included in the study was paired according to age (± 1year), socio-economic status and primiparity with a Greek woman that gave birth the same time period in the same maternity ward. In order to avoid selection bias the women were paired in chronological order so the first ethnic Albanian woman who was included in the study was matched with the first suitable Greek women who agreed to participate in the study and so on. To define the women socio-economic status the Madianos and Zarnari Social and Economical Status Scale was used (Madianos and Zarnari, 1988). According to this scale, women were grouped into three major categories: low (farmers, labourers and blue collar workers), medium (technicians, self-employed persons, medium employees, small and medium sized shop owners) and upper status (scientists, executives, high ranking corporate employees). Primiparity was selected as a matching variable because results from earlier studies showed a correlation of primiparity with the manifestation of maternity blues

(Pop et al, 1995). It should be noted though that newer studies did not report similar results (Hay and Levy, 2003, Gonidakis et al, 2007).

### 4.1.2 Data collection

Demographic and clinical data concerning pregnancy, delivery and puerperium were collected by questionnaire as well as from the women's medical records.

The first day after delivery all women were asked to complete the State Trait Anxiety Inventory (Spielberger et al, 1970) and the List of Threatening Experience (Brugha et al, 1985) for the period of pregnancy. All the above questionnaires were self-administered. Finally the Montgomery Asberg Depression Rating Scale (Montgomery and Asberg, 1979) was completed by the author following a 20 minutes face-to-face interview during which the participants's emotional status during the last month was discussed.

All women were asked to complete the Kennerley and Gath (1989) Blues Questionnaire every evening for the first 3 days following delivery. The face-to-face interviews were limited to the first 3 days of puerperium as this was the minimum time that the women stayed in the hospital after delivery. Although the above questionnaires were self-administered the author was always available to offer assistance on the scale's questions.

At the end of the 1st month and 3rd month all women were interviewed by telephone. During these interviews the Edinburgh Postnatal Depression Scale (Cox et al, 1987) was administered. We also recorded whether the women were breastfeeding, and if according to their judgment their babies were crying a lot and/or having a poor sleep.

In the case of a participant reporting symptoms of depression further psychiatric evaluation was suggested. All women gave written informed consent in order to participate in the study and they provided the author with their telephone numbers in order to reach them after their discharge from the maternity ward

### 4.1.3 Measures

For the purposes of the study the following measures were used:

a. Blues Questionnaire (Kennerley and Gath, 1989) was used to measure maternity blues. The Blues Questionnaire (BQ) is a validated self-rating scale consisting of 28 questions concerning the emotional state after delivery. The available answers are "yes" or "no" so the maximum score is 28 and the minimum 0. For the calculation of the cut-off point for severe maternity blues the authors suggest that the mean peak score of all women should be used. The highest score on any of the days of observation is considered the peak score for each participant. For the present study the mean peak score was 8.4 so the cut off point for the diagnosis of severe maternity blues was the score of 9. It should be noted that the B.Q. was translated, back translated and adapted in Greek for the purposes of a previous study on maternity blues (Gonidakis et al, 2007).
b. The Edinburgh Postnatal Depression Scale (EPDS) was produced by Cox et al, (1987). It consists of 10 items with four possible answers for each item. The score for each item varies from 0 to 3 so the maximum score is 30. The EPDS has been translated in many languages and used worldwide as a reliable screening instrument for postnatal

depression (Gibson et al, 2009, Halbreich and Karkun, 2006). The validation of the Greek edition of EPDS was conducted by Leonardou et al (2009) who calculated the cut off point for the diagnosis of postnatal depression at 11/12. When the Greek version of EPDS was administered together with SCID, it produced a sensitivity of 90% and a specificity of 97.22% (Leonardou et al, 2009). For the present study a cut off point of 12 was used.

c. Montgomery-Asberg Depression Rating Scale (MADRS) (Montgomery and Asberg, 1979) is a semi structured 10item scale. The MADRS focuses more on the psychic manifestations of depression rather on the somatic ones and thus is more suitable for the measurement of depression in women that due to pregnancy and delivery are experiencing a lot of somatic disturbances that resemble the somatic symptoms of depression. The MADRS have been translated, back translated and adjusted in Greek by other research groups in University of Athens.
d. The List of Threatening Experience (L.T.E.) is a 12item scale of stressful life events created by Brugha et al (1985) that have been used successfully in puerpartum studies (Gonidakis 2007, 2008; Yamashita et al, 2000). The same procedure that was followed with the B.Q. for the translation and adjustment of the scale in the Greek language has also been followed with LTE
e. The State-Trait Anxiety Inventory (STAI) is a widely used self rating scale produced by Spielberger et al (1970) that consists of two 20 items subscales measuring anxiety as state and trait. The scale has been translated and validated for the Greek language (Liakos and Gianitsi, 1984)
f. Demographic and clinical data concerning pregnancy, delivery and puerpartum were collected by questionnaire as well as from the participant's medical records

### 4.1.4 Analysis

Chi-square was used to compare nominal variables. Two-tailed paired samples t-test was used to compare mean scores of scale variables between the Albanian and Greek group. A Kolmogorov-Smirnov Z test was run prior to the analysis to detect differences in the locations and shapes of the distributions between the two groups measurements. Since the test did not show any significant differences in BQ 3rd day ($Z=0.5$, $p= 0.9$), EPDS 1st month ($Z=0.7$, $p= 0.8$), or MADRS ($Z=0.8$, $p=0.6$) distributions paired samples t-test was performed. One way Analysis of Variance (ANOVA) test was used, to compare the daily BQ scores between immigrant and Greek women in the Maternity Blues and non Maternity Blues group as well as the EPDS scores between immigrant and Greek women in the Postpartum Depression and non Postpartum Depression group. Forward binary logistic regression analysis was used to further investigate factors that differentiate the two national groups as well as to investigate factors that were related with maternity blues and postpartum depression in immigrant women. Also for each regression analysis a Hosmer-Lemeshow test was run in order to test whether the model produced by regression analysis has goodness of fit. Finally the value of Nagelkerkle R square was calculated as an indication of the predictability of the model produced by regression analysis.

The research design was approved by the relevant ethical and scientific committee of University of Athens, Medical School, 1st Department of Psychiatry.

### 4.2 Results

Twenty-two of the total 100 immigrant women were excluded from the study leading to a response rate of 78%. Nine of the 22 women (40.9%) could not speak and/or read Greek, 5 (22.7%) refused to participate and 1 (4.5%) was found suffering from depression in day 1 (MADRS >20). Seven (31.9 %) immigrant women could not be matched with a Greek counterpart so they were excluded from the study. In addition 5 Greek women refused to participate in the study and 2 were excluded because the were suffering from depression in day 1 after delivery. The sample characteristics are summarized in table 1:

| Variables | | Immigrant | | Greek | |
|---|---|---|---|---|---|
| Demographic and social | | F | % | F | % |
| Age | 18-20 | 6 | 7.7% | 7 | 5.1% |
| | 21-25 | 32 | 41% | 27 | 34.6% |
| | 26-30 | 27 | 34.6% | 30 | 38.5% |
| | >30 | 13 | 16.7% | 14 | 21.8% |
| Education Level | Primary | 8 | 10.3% | 6 | 7.7% |
| | Secondary | 55 | 70.5% | 53 | 68% |
| | Tertiary | 15 | 19.2% | 19 | 24.3% |
| Marital status | Married | 75 | 96.2% | 76 | 97.4% |
| Years of marriage | 1-5 | 56 | 71.8% | 62 | 79.5% |
| | >5 | 22 | 28.2% | 16 | 20.5% |
| Socio-economic Status | Low | 59 | 75.7% | 59 | 75.7% |
| | Medium | 18 | 23.1% | 18 | 23.1% |
| | Upper | 1 | 1.3% | 1 | 1.3% |
| Residence in Greece | 1year | 1 | 1.3% | | |
| | 2-5 years | 54 | 69.2% | | |
| | >5 years | 23 | 29.5% | | |
| Occupation | Working | 52 | 66.7% | 48 | 61.5% |
| Pregnancy and delivery | | | | | |
| Abortions | 0 | 71 | 91% | 64 | 82.1% |
| | >1 | 7 | 9% | 14 | 17.9% |
| Primiparity | yes | 46 | | | 59,00% |
| Unwanted pregnancy | Yes | 7 | 9% | 16 | 20.5% |
| Method of delivery | Natural birth | 53 | 67.9% | 44 | 56.4% |
| | Ceasarotomy | 25 | 32.1% | 34 | 43.6% |
| Puerperium | | | | | |
| Intention to breastfeed | Yes | 75 | 96.2% | 69 | 88.5% |
| Support from family | Yes | 41 | 52.6% | 51 | 65.4% |
| Advice | Yes | 53 | 67.9% | 66 | 84.6% |
| Peer support | Yes | 49 | 62.8% | 48 | 61.5% |

Table 1. Sample characteristics. F: frequency

#### 4.2.1 Differences between immigrant and Greek women

The two groups of women were quite similar. When they were compared to each other only two differences emerged. The first was that immigrant women reported lower number of abortions than Greek women (p=0.04) (table 1&2). The second was that lower number of immigrant women reported that they would be able to consult a family member or friend or issues concerning rearing the child (p=0.01) (table 1&3).

| Variables | Immigrant N=78 | | Greek N=78 | | Paired samples t-test | | |
|---|---|---|---|---|---|---|---|
| | mean | sd | mean | sd | t | df | p |
| Demographic and social | | | | | | | |
| Years of marriage | 4.2 | 3.2 | 3.6 | 3.3 | 1.3 | 77 | 0.2 |
| Years of education | 12 | 1.9 | 11.5 | 2.6 | 1.4 | 77 | 0.2 |
| Medical | | | | | | | |
| Number of abortions | 0.1 | 0.3 | 0.2 | 0.5 | 2 | 77 | 0.04 |
| Number of stillbirths | 0.2 | 0.5 | 0.2 | 0.3 | 1.1 | 77 | 0.3 |
| Clinical Measurements | | | | | | | |
| MADRS 1st day | 6 | 5,9 | 6,8 | 5,6 | 10.9 | 77 | 0.3 |
| STAI trait | 29.1 | 6.1 | 28.8 | 7.4 | 0.2 | 77 | 0.8 |
| STAI state | 31.3 | 7.3 | 33.9 | 9.5 | 1.6 | 77 | 0.1 |
| LTE | 1.2 | 1.2 | 1.5 | 1.2 | 1.5 | 77 | 0.2 |

sd: standard deviation, df: degrees of freedom, p:level of significance

Table 2. Comparison between immigrant and Greek women. Scale variables

| Variables | Chi Square | | |
|---|---|---|---|
| N=156 | $X^2$ | df | p |
| Demographic and social | | | |
| Marital status | 0.2 | 1 | 0.6 |
| Employment status | 0.5 | 1 | 0.5 |
| Pregnancy and delivery | | | |
| Unwanted pregnancy | 3.5 | 1 | 0.06 |
| Method of delivery | 2.2 | 1 | 0.1 |
| Puerperium | | | |
| Intention to breastfeed | 3.3 | 1 | 0.07 |
| Support from family | 2.7 | 1 | 0.1 |
| Advice on upbringing the child | 6 | 1 | 0.01 |
| Peer support | 0.03 | 1 | 0.9 |

df: degrees of freedom, p:level of significance

Table 3. Comparison between immigrant and Greek women. Nominal variables

### 4.2.2 Maternity blues

When the cut-off point of 9 was applied, 13 (16.7%) of the 78 immigrant and 14 (17.9%) of the 78 Greek women experienced maternity blues the 1st day after delivery. Accordingly, 12 (15.4%) immigrant and 14 (17.9%) Greek women experienced maternity blues the 2nd day after delivery and finally 17 (21.8%) immigrant and 19 (24.4%) Greek women experienced maternity blues the 3rd day after delivery. During the first three days after delivery 18

(23.1%) immigrant and 27 (34.6%) Greek women in total experienced maternity blues. There was no statistical significant difference between the two groups considering the percentage of the women that developed maternity blues in each and any of the three days of puerperium (table 4)

| Variables | Chi Square | | |
|---|---|---|---|
| N=156 | $X^2$ | df | p |
| 1st day | 0.45 | 1 | 0.8 |
| 2nd day | 0.2 | 1 | 0.7 |
| 3rd day | 0.1 | 1 | 0.7 |
| Any of the 3 days of observation | 2.5 | 1 | 0.1 |

sd: standard deviation, df: degrees of freedom, p:level of significance

Table 4. Comparison between immigrant and Greek women that developed Maternity Blues

The daily fluctuation of the BQ score in the group of women who developed maternity blues and in the group of women who did not develop maternity blues in any of the three days of observation is represented in figure 1.

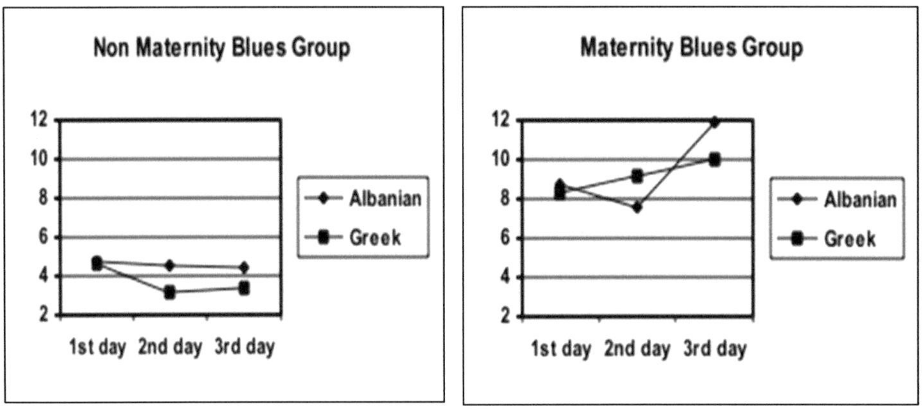


Fig. 1. Daily BQ's mean score variation in both the Maternity Blues and non Maternity Blues Groups

The comparison of the daily BQ scores between immigrant and Greek women in the Maternity Blues group did not show any difference. The comparison of the daily BQ scores in the non-Maternity Blues group showed higher scores for the immigrant group during the 2nd (p: 0.001) and 3rd day (p: 0.02) measurements (table 5).

Forward stepwise logistic regression analysis was used in order to confirm the findings for the Maternity Blues and non Maternity Blues groups. The BQ score for each day together with MADRS score, number of abortions and consultation on rearing the child (categorical variable) were entered as independent variables. For the MB group no difference was found between immigrant and Greek women. For the non MB group 2nd day BQ score (p: 0.01, odds ratio: 1.4) and consultation on rearing the child (p: 0.05, odd ratio: 0.4) were the two factors that could differentiate immigrant and Greek women thus verifying that even when the two demographic differences between Albanian and Greek women were taken into consideration maternity blues symptomatology was still more severe during the 2nd day after delivery in the group of immigrant women that did not experience maternity blues. The significance level of the Hosmer-Lemeshow test (p:0.4) and the value of Nagelkerkle R square (0.18) indicate that the model produced by regression analysis has goodness of fit, and it can predict around 18% of nationality variance.

| Variables | One way ANOVA | |
|---|---|---|
| | F | p |
| Maternity Blues group | | |
| 1st day | 0.09 | 0.8 |
| 2nd day | 1,2 | 0.3 |
| 3rd day | 2,6 | 0.1 |
| Non Maternity Blues group | | |
| 1st day | 0.1 | 0.9 |
| 2nd day | 11,4 | 0.01 |
| 3rd day | 6,1 | 0.02 |

Table 5. Blues Questionnaire daily score. Comparison between immigrant and Greek women in the Maternity Blues and non-Maternity Blues group. One Way Analysis of Variance with Bonferoni correction. p: level of significance

To explore further the factors that could be related to the manifestation of maternity blues in immigrant women a second stepwise logistic regression was conducted. The age, years of education, months of residence in Greece, years of marriage, social-economic status as well as the STAI, MADRS and LTE scores were entered as independent variables. The only difference between the immigrant women that developed maternity blues during the three days of observation and those that did not was the STAI state anxiety (p: 0.001, odds ratio: 1.2). The result indicate that immigrant women who were more anxious immediately after delivery were more likely to develop maternity blues. The significance level of the Hosmer-Lemeshow test (p:0.5) and the value of Nagelkerkle R square (0.29) indicate that the model produced by regression analysis has goodness of fit, and it can predict around 29% of the maternity blues manifestation in immigrant women.

### 4.2.3 Postpartum depression

Sixty eight of the 78 (87.2%) immigrant women and 74 of the original 78 (94.9%) Greek women were reached at 1st month telephone interview. Eight (11,8%) immigrant and 10 Greek (13,5%) women had EPDS scores greater than 12. Sixty five of the 78 (83.3%) immigrant women and 68 of the 78 (87.2%) Greek women were reached at 3rd month telephone interview. Nine immigrant (11,6%) and 8 (11,6%) Greek women had EPDS scores greater that 12. Overall 11 (15,7%) of the immigrant women and 15 (20,3%) of the Greek women scored higher than 12 in the EPDS in either or both the 1st and 3rd months measurements. The comparison of the two groups did not show any statistically significant difference (table 6).

The comparison of the EPDS scores between immigrant and Greek women in the Postpartum Depression group did not show any difference. Similarly, absence of any difference in the EPDS score between immigrant and Greek women was also observed in the non-Postpartum Depression group (table 7).

| Variables | Chi Square | | |
|---|---|---|---|
| N=156 | $X^2$ | df | p |
| 1st month | 0.9 | 1 | 0.8 |
| 3rd month | 0.9 | 1 | 0.8 |
| Any of the 2 interviews | 0.5 | 1 | 0.5 |

sd: standard deviation, df: degrees of freedom, p:level of significance

Table 6. Comparison between immigrant and Greek women that developed Postpartum depressive symptomatology.

| Variables | One way ANOVA | |
|---|---|---|
| | F | p |
| Postpartum Depression group | | |
| 1st month | 0.9 | 0.4 |
| 3rd month | 3.7 | 0.07 |
| Non Postpartum Depression group | | |
| 1st day | 0.001 | 0.9 |
| 2nd day | 0.02 | 0.9 |

Table 7. EDPS scores. Comparison between immigrant and Greek women in the Postpartum Depression and non-Postpartum Depression group. One Way Analysis of Variance with Bonferoni correction. p: level of significance

Forward stepwise logistic regression analysis was used in order to confirm the findings for the Postpartum Depression and non Postpartum Depression groups. The EPDS score for each day together with MADRS, LTE, STAI scores, number of abortions and consultation on rearing the child (categorical variable) were entered as independent variables. For the Postpartum Depression group 3rd month score (p: 0.07, odds ratio: 1.2) was the only factor that could differentiate immigrant and Greek women. The significance level of the Hosmer-Lemeshow test (p:0.4) and the value of Nagelkerkle R square (0.32) indicate that the model produced by regression analysis has goodness of fit, and it can predict around 32% of nationality variance. For the non-Postpartum Depression group no difference was found between immigrant and Greek women.

To explore further the factors that could be related to the manifestation of Postpartum Depression symptomatology in immigrant women a second stepwise logistic regression was conducted. The age, years of education, months of residence in Greece, years of marriage, social-economic status and the manifestation of Maternity Blues as well as the STAI, MADRS, LTE scores were entered as independent variables. The only difference between the immigrant women that developed Postpartum Depressive symptomatology and those that did not was the STAI trait anxiety (p: 0.001, odds ratio: 1.1). The result indicate that immigrant women who had more anxious personality traits were more likely to develop Postpartum Depression symptomatology. The significance level of the Hosmer-Lemeshow test (p:0.2) and the value of Nagelkerkle R square (0.54) indicate that the model produced by regression analysis has goodness of fit, and it can predict around 54% of the EPDS variance.

### 4.3 Discussion

The two matched groups showed very few differences in the statistical analysis. The first difference concerned family planning, that is the number of abortions. Greek women have one of the highest rates of abortions in Europe and very low prevalence of contraceptive use apart from withdrawal and condoms (Ioannidi-Kapolou, 2004). The above findings could explain the differences in family planning between the two ethnic groups.

The second difference between the two groups concerned the level of support and especially the availability of consultation on issues of child rearing. Although the Albanian community is the largest immigrant community in Greece, more Albanian women replied that they did not have someone to consult or that they would not be helped during the first month of puerperium (the latter was not statistically significant).

Regarding the first aim of the study, that is to explore possible differences in the manifestation of maternity blues and postpartum depression between immigrant and mainstream culture women the results showed that very few differences existed between the two groups. A first difference was that immigrant women that did not fully develop maternity blues reported more maternity blues symptoms during the 2nd and 3rd day after delivery than Greek women. Logistic regression analysis confirmed that 2nd day symptomatology in the non Maternity Blues group was more severe in the immigrant women who also felt that they did not have adequate advice on rearing their child. The above result lead us to the conclusion that a number of immigrant women might be experiencing a more severe sub threshold type of maternity blues than Greek women. Although Kumar (1994) in his review on the relation between postnatal mental illness and transcultural factors suggested that maternity blues: "does not appear in a major way to be related to environmental, social or cultural factors", it seems, however, that some variations might exist in the expression of mild maternity blues symptomatology among women from different cultures.

A second possible difference was found in the 3rd month EPDS scores in the group of women that developed postpartum depression symptomatology. The Greek women seemed to have higher EPDS scores than the immigrant women. It should be noted that this difference did not reach statistical significance either in the ANOVA or the logistic regression analysis so it not possible to draw a definite conclusion on this result.

Contrary to the study's original hypothesis the results indicate that there are no major differences in the prevalence of postpartum depression symptomatology and maternity blues between immigrant and Greek mothers. This result is in accordance with other studies that did not find that immigration status had an impact on postpartum depression rates (Kuo et al, 2004), especially in majority immigrant groups (Mechakra-Tahiri et al, 2007; Zelkowitz et al, 2008). A possible explanation for this result is the role of social factors (Bandyopadhyay, 2010; Steward et al, 2008; Taniguchi and Baruffi, 2009) and adjustment to the mainstream culture (Gonidakis et al, 2011) in the development of depressive symptomatology. The immigrant women that participated in the study had similar socio-economical status to the Greek women, they were part of the largest immigrant group in Greece, 98.7% of them had been living in Greece more than one year, 66.7% replied that they had a steady job, and 81.3% had insurance coverage. Furthermore their country of origin, Albania, shares borders with Greece and it not uncommon for relatives to travel from one country to the other in order to visit their kin. The study results could be used cautiously to confirm the suggestion that the impact of immigration in the development of postpartum depression is mediated through lack of support and socio-economical adversities. The comparison between immigrant and Greek women did not produce major differences in the rates of maternity blues and postnatal depression symptomatology probably because these factors did not differ greatly between the two groups.

Considering the second aim of the study, to explore possible factors that influence the manifestation of maternity blues and postpartum depression in immigrants, anxiety was the main factor that was produced from the analysis of the research data. It is interesting that according to the study's results anxiety after delivery (state anxiety) was related to the development of maternity blues while anxiety as a personality characteristic (trait anxiety) was related to the development of postpartum depression symptomatology. The relation between anxiety and depression is well established in the literature (Pollack, 2005). Specifically in the period of puerperium prenatal and antenatal anxiety has been related to the development of postpartum depression (Heron et al, 2004; Skouteris et al, 2009). Similar relation has been found between maternity blues and anxiety disorders in the puerperium (Gonidakis et al, 2007; Reck et al, 2009). It is noteworthy that contrary to various reports in the literature stressful life events during pregnancy were not related to either maternity blues or postpartum depression symptomatology (Collins et al, 2011; Gonidakis et al, 2008).

The main limitations of the study were three. Firstly the immigrant sample was restricted to one hospital and to women from Albania that had an adequate knowledge of Greek. The result of the above restriction was that the study included women who might have had a better adjustment in Greece than women who were excluded from the study and can not be generalized to the whole immigrant population. On the other hand only 9 out of 100 immigrant women were excluded from the study because of language difficulties. One explanation for the above is that immigrant Albanian women decide to have a child in Greece after a few years in the country and by that time they would have learned the language, acquired staying permission, steady employment and insurance coverage. The second limitation of the study was that the questionnaires were administered in Greek. Although all immigrant women could read Greek they still faced some difficulties understanding some of the questions. An effort was made to counteract the above difficulty with the presence of the author who could offer assistance with the scales' questions. The third limitation was that the study's design did not enable to obtain data from the fourth and fifth day of puerperium who are also crucial for the development of maternity blues (Hau and Levy, 2003; Hensaw, 2003; Rodhe et al, 1997) Thus the prevalence, time patterns and symptomatology reported in this study describe only the first three days and no conclusion can be drawn for the whole period that maternity blues last.

In conclusion the study's results indicate that there are only minor differences in the manifestation of maternity blues and postpartum depression between Albanian immigrant and Greek women. The two more interesting findings were that there might be a percentage of immigrant women that suffer from a more severe sub threshold type of maternity blues and also that anxiety seems to be the factor related with maternity blues and postpartum depression symptomatology in immigrants.

## 5. Conclusion

Immigrant women face a number of adversities that may compromise their mental health especially during the sensitive period after delivery. Difficulties comprehending and adapting to everyday life in a new environment, their wish to gain acceptance and safety in their host country, the lack of support and the transition from the heritage to the mainstream meaning of motherhood and finally, their struggle to "forget" traumatizing experience and make a "fresh start" in a new place are some of the issues commonly discussed by immigrant mothers. Although some of these issues may be related to the deterioration of maternal mood during the puerperium no conclusive evidence can be drawn from the available reports in the literature. Lack of support, stressful life events during pregnancy and anxiety seem to be three of the factors that are related with maternity blues and postpartum depression in immigrants. However, there is still a gap of knowledge on the interplay between culture, spirituality, acculturation and women's mood during this sensitive period. Furthermore the methodological difficulties in transcultural research hamper the expansion of our knowledge on maternity blues and postpartum depression in immigrant population.

The health worker's awareness of the relationship between immigration and mood disorders and their efforts to facilitate women's adaptation to the new situation can have a positive impact on the new mother's mental health. Of course, additional factors such as pre-immigration circumstances and the role of local ethnic communities should also be examined in order to obtain a more comprehensive view of the manifestation of postpartum depression and maternity blues in immigrant women.

## 6. Acknowledgments

Special thanks go to Emeritus Professor of Psychiatry A. Rabavilas, Emeritus Professor of Psychiatry G.N. Christodoulou, Professor of Gynecology G. Kreatsas and Associate Professor E. Varsou for their invaluable help in the preparation and conduct of the research that was presented in this chapter. Also to Mis E. Rogakou for her support with statistical analysis of the study's results and S. Zoakos MPhil and M. Anyfantaki MSc for proofreading the manuscript.

## 7. References

Abbott, MW. & Williams, MM., (2006). Postnatal depressive symptoms among Pacific mothers in Auckland: prevalence and risk factors. *Australian and New Zealand Journal of Psychiatry*. Vol. 40, No. 3, pp. 230-238.

Affonso, DD.; De, AK.; Horowitz, JA. and Mayberry LJ., (2000). An international study exploring levels of postpartum depressive symptomatology. *Journal of Psychosomatic Research*. Vol. 49, No 3, pp. 207-216.

Bale, TL., (2006). Stress, sensitivity and the development of affective disorders. *Hormones and Behavior*, Vol. 50, No. 4, pp. 529–533.

Bandyopadhyay, M.; Small, R.; Watson, LF. and Brown, S., (2010). Life with a new baby: how do immigrant and Australian-born women's experiences compare? *Australian and New Zealand Journal of Public Health*. Vol.34, No 4, pp. 412-421.

Beck, CT.; Froman, RD. and Bernal, H., (2005). Acculturation level and postpartum depression in Hispanic mothers. *MCN the American Journal of Maternal Child Nursing*. Vol. 30, No. 5, pp. 299-304.

Beck, CT., (2001). Predictors of postpartum depression: an update. *Nursing Research*. Vol. 50, pp. 275-285

Bergant, AM.; Heim, K.; Ulmer, H. and Illmensee, K., (1999). Early postnatal depressive : associations with obstestric and psychosocial factors. *Journal of Psychosomatic Research*. Vol. 46, No. 4, pp.391-394.

Berry, JW., (2006). Stress perspectives on acculturation. In: *The Cambridge handbook of acculturation psychology,* Sam, D. and & Berry JW., pp. 43-57, Cambridge University Press, Cambridge.

Berry, JW., (1980). Acculturation as varieties of adaptation. In: *Acculturation: Theory, models and some findings,* Padilla A, pp. 9-25, Boulder, CO, Westview.

Bhugra, D., (2003). Migration and depression. *Acta Psychiatrica Scandinavia,* Vol. 418(suppl) pp. 62–67.

Bhugra, D., (2004a). Migration, distress and cultural identity. *British Medical Bulletin,* Vol. 69, pp. 29–141.

Bhugra, D., (2004b). Migration and Mental Health. *Acta Psychiatrica Scandinavia,* Vol. 109, pp. 243–258.

Bhui, K. and Bhugra, D., (2001). Transcultural psychiatry: Some social and epidemiological research issues. *International Journal of Social Psychiatry*, Vol. 47, No. 3, pp.1–9.

Bjerke, SE.; Vangen, S.; Nordhagen, R.; Ytterdahl, T.; Magnus, P. and Stray-Pedersen, B., (2008). Postpartum depression among Pakistani women in Norway: prevalence and risk factors. *The Journal of Maternal-Fetal and Neonatal Medicine*. Vol. 21, No. 12, pp. 889-94.

Brugha, T.; Bebbington, P.; Tennant, C. and Hurry, J., (1985). The list of threatening experiences: a subset of 12 life event categories with considerable long term contextual threat. *Psychological Medicine*, Vol.15, pp. 189-194.

Collins, CH.; Zimmerman, C. and Howard, LM., (2011). Refugee, asylum seeker, immigrant women and postnatal depression: rates and risk factors. *Archives of Women Mental Health.* Vol 14, No. 1, pp. 3-11.

Cox, JL.; Holden, JM. and Sagovsky, R., (1987). Detection of postnatal depression: development of the 10-item Edinburgh Postnatal Depression Scale. *British Journal of Psychiatry*. Vol. 150, pp. 782-786

Daher,AM.; Ibrahim, H.;, Daher, TM. and Anbori, AK., (2011). Health related quality of life among Iraqi immigrants settled in Malaysia. *BMC Public Health.* Vol. 30, No. 11, pp. 407

Darcy, JM.; Grzywacz, JG.; Stephens, RL.; Leng, I.; Clinch, CR. and Arcury, TA.; (2011). Maternal depressive symptomatology: 16 mont follow-up of infent and maternal health-related quality of life. *Journal of the American Board of Family Medicine*, Vol. 24, No. 3, pp. 249-257.

Davila, M.; McFall, SL. and Cheng, D., (2009). Acculturation and depressive symptoms among pregnant and postpartum Latinas. *Maternal and Child Health Journal.* Vol.13, No. 3, pp. 318-325.

Fung, K. and Dennis, CL., (2010). Postpartum depression among immigrant women. *Current Opinion in Psychiatry*, Vol.23, No 4, pp. 342-348.

Foss, GF. (2001). Maternal sensitivity, posttraumatic stress, and acculturation in Vietnamese and Hmong mothers. *MCN. The American Journal of Maternal and Child Nursing*. Vol. 26, No.5, pp. 257-263.

Gibson, J.; McKenzie-McHarg, K.; Shakespeare, J.; Price, J. and Gray, RA., (2009). A systematic review of studies validating the Edinburgh Postnatal Depression Scale in antepartum and postpartum women.*Acta Psychiatrica Scandinavia*. Vol.119, No. 5, pp. 350-364.

Gonidakis, F.; Korakakis, P.; Ploubidis, D.; Karapavlou, DA.; Rogakou, E. and Madianos, M., (2011). The relationship between acculturation factors and symptoms of depression: A cross-sectional study with immigrants living in Athens. *Transcultural Psychiatry*, vol. 48, No. 4, pp. 437-454.

Gonidakis, F.; Rabavilas, AD.; Varsou, E.; Kreatsas, G. and Christodoulou, GN., (2008). A 6 month study of postpartum depression and related factors in Athens Greece. *Comprehensive Psychiatry*, Vol. 49, No. 3, pp. 275-282.

Gonidakis, F.; Rabavilas, AD.; Varsou, E.; Kreatsas, G. and Christodoulou, GN., (2007). Maternity blues in Athens, Greece: a study during the first 3 days after delivery. *Journal of Affective Disorders*, Vol. 99, No. 1-3, pp. 107-115.

Grigoriadis, S,; Erlick Robinson, G.; Fung, K.; Ross, LE.; Chee, CY.; Dennis, CL. and Romans, S., (2009). Traditional postpartum practices and rituals: clinical implications. *Canadian Journal of Psychiatry*. Vol. 54, No. 12, pp. 834-840.

Gross, R.; Brammli-Greenberg, S. and Remennick, L., (2001). Self-rated health status and health care utilization among immigrant and non-immigrant Israeli Jewish women. *Women Health*. Vol. 34, No.3, pp. 53-69.

Halbreich, U. and Karkun, S., (2006). Cross-cultural and social diversity of prevalence of postpartum depression and depressive symptoms. *Journal of Affective Disorders*. Vol. 91, No 2-3, pp. 97-111.

Harris, B., (1981). Maternity Blues in East African Clinic Attenders. *Archives of General Psychiatry*. Vol. 38, pp. 1293-1295.

Hau, F. and Levy, V., (2003). The maternity blues and Hong-Kong Chinese women: an exploratory study. *Journal of Affective Disorders*. Vol. 75, pp. 197-203.

Hensaw, C., (2003). Mood disturbances in the early puerperium. a review. *Archives of Women Mental Health*. Vol. 6, suppl2, pp.33-42.

Heron, J.; O'Connor, TG.; Evans, J.; Golding, J. and Glover, V.; ALSPAC Study Team (2004). The course of anxiety and depression through pregnancy and the postpartum in a community sample. *Journal of Affective Disorders*. Vol. 80, No. 1, pp. 65-73.

Huang, YC. and Mathers, NJ., (2008). Postnatal depression and the experience of South Asian marriage migrant women in Taiwan: survey and semi-structured interview study. *International Journal of Nursing Studies*. Vol. 45, No. 6, pp. 924-931.

Hull, D., (1979). Migration, adaptation, and illness: a review. *Social Science and Medicine. Medical Psychology and Medical Sociology*. Vol. 13A, No. 1, pp. 25-36.

Ioannidi-Kapolou, E., (2004). Use of contraception and abortion in Greece: a review. *Reproductive and Health Matters*. Vol. 12, No. 24 suppl, pp.174-183.

Kennerley, H. and Gath, D., (1989). Maternity blues. I. Detection and measurement by questionnaire. *British Journal of Psychiatry*. Vol. 155, pp. 356-62.

Kumar, R., (1994). Post natal mental illness: a transcultural perspective. *Social Psychiatry and Psychiatric Epidemiology*. Vol 29, No. 6, pp. 250-264.

Kuo, WH.; Wilson, TE.; Holman, S.; Fuentes-Afflick, E.; O'Sullivan, MJ. and Minkoff, H., (2004). Depressive symptoms in the immediate postpartum period among Hispanic women in three U.S. Cities. *Journal of Immigrants Health*. Vol. 6, No. 4, pp. 145-53.

La Fromboise, T.; Coleman, HLK. and Gerton, J., (1993). Psychological impact of biculturism: Evidence and theory. *Psychological Bulletin*, Vol. 114, pp. 395–412.

Leonardou, AA.; Zervas, YM.; Papageorgiou, CC.; Marks, MN.; Tsartsara, EC.; Antsaklis, A.; Christodoulou, GN. and Soldatos, CR., (2009). Validation of the Edinburgh Postnatal Depression Scale and prevalence of postnatal depression at two months postpartum in a sample of Greek mothers. *Journal of Reproductive and Infant Psychology* Vol. 27, No. 1, pp. 28-39.

Liakos, A. and Giannitsia S., (1984). The validity of the revised Greek Spielberger State Trait Anxiety Inventory. *Encefalos*. Vol.21, pp. 71-76 (in Greek).

Lindert, J.; Schouler-Ocak, M.; Heinz, A. and Priebe, S.; (2008). Mental health, health care utilisation of migrants in Europe.*European Psychiatry*. Vol.23 Suppl 1, pp.14-20.

Nagata, M.; Nagai, Y.; Sobajima, H.; Ando, T.; Nishide, Y. and Honjo, S.; (2000). Maternity blues and attachment to children in mothers of full term normal infants. *Acta Psychiatrica Scandinavia*. Vol. 101, No 3, pp. 209-217.

Madianos, MG.; Gonidakis, F.; Ploubidis, D.; Papadopoulou, E. and Rogakou, E., (2008). Measuring acculturation and symptoms of depression of foreign immigrants in the Athens area. *International Journal of Social Psychiatry*. Vol. 54, No. 4, pp. 338-349.

Madianos, M. and Zarnari, O., (1988). Indicator of socio-economic status. In: *Health and Greek society*. pp. 28-30, National Center of Social Research, Athens, Greece.

Mann, R.; Gilbody, S. and Adamson, J., (2010). Prevalence and incidence of postnatal depression: what can systematic reviews tell us? *Archives of Womens Mental Health*. Vol. 13, No 4, pp.295-305.

Mechakra-Tahiri, S.; Zunzunegui, MV. and Seguin, L., (2007). Self-rated health and postnatal depressive symptoms among immigrant mothers in Québec. *Women Health*. Vol. 45, No. 4, pp. 1-17.

Mirsky, J.; Kohn, R.; Levav, I.; Grinshpoon, A. and Ponizovsky, AM.; (2008). Psychological distress and common mental disorders among immigrants: results from the Israeli based component of the world mental health survey. *Journal of Clinical Psychiatry*. Vol. 69, No. 11, pp. 1715-1720.

Miszkurka, M.; Goulet, L. and Zunzunegui, MV., (2010). Contributions of immigration to depressive symptoms among pregnant women in Canada. *Canadian Journal of Public Health*. Vol. 101, No. 5, pp. 358-64.

Moloney, J., (1952). Post partum depression or third day depression following childbirth. *New Orleans Child and Parent Digest*. Vol. 6, pp.20-32.

Montgomery, SA. and Asberg, M., (1977). A new depression scale designed to be sensitive to change. *British Journal of Psychiatry*. Vol. 134, pp. 382-389.

Morrow, M.; Smith, JE.; Lai, Y. and Jaswal, S., (2008). Shifting landscapes: immigrant women and postpartum depression. *Health Care of Women International*. Vol. 29, No. 6, pp. 593-61.

Murata, A.; Nadaoka, T.; Morioka, Y.; Oiji, A. and Saito, H., (1998). Prevalence and background factors of maternity blues. *Gynecologic and Obstetric Investigation*. Vol. 46, pp. 99-104.

Nguyen, HT.; Clark, M. and Ruiz, RJ., (2007). Effects of acculturation on the reporting of depressive symptoms among Hispanic pregnant women. *Nursing Research*, Vol, 56, No 3, pp. 217–223.

Nagata, M.; Nagai, Y.; Sobajima, H.; Ando, T.; Nishide, Y. and Honjo, S., (2000). Maternity blues and attachment to children in mothers of full-term normal infants. *Acta Psychiatrica Scandinavica,* Vol. 101, No. 3, pp. 209-217

O'Hara, M.; Schlechte, J.; Lewis, D. and Wright, E., (1991). Prospective study of postpartum blues. *Archives of General Psychiatry.* Vol. 48, pp.801-806.

Ozeki, N., (2008). Transcultural stress factors of Japanese mothers living in the United Kingdom. *Journal of Transcultural Nursing*. Vol.19, No. 1, pp. 47-54.

Pitt, B., (1973). Maternity Blues. *British Journal of Psychiatry*. Vol. 122, pp. 431-433. Pollack, MH., (2005). Comorbid anxiety and depression. *Journal of Clinical Psychiatry*. Vol. 66, No. 8 (Suppl), pp. 22-29.

Pop, VJ.; Wijnen, HA.; Van Montfort, M.; Essed, GG.; De Geus, CA.; Van Son, MM. and Komproe, IH., (1995). Blues and depression during early puerperium: home versus hospital deliveries. *British Journal of Obstetrics and Gynaecology*. Vol.102, pp. 701-706.

Reck, C.; Stehle, E.; Reinig, K. and Mundt, C., (2009). Maternity blues as a predictor of DSM-IV depression and anxiety disorders in the first three months postpartum. *Journal of Affective Disorders* Vol. 113, No. 1-2, pp. 77-87.

Robertson, E.; Grace, S.; Wallington, T. and Stewart, DE., (2004). Antenatal risk factors for postpartum depression: a synthesis of recent literature. *General Hospital Psychiatry*. Vol. 26, No. 4, pp. 289-295.

Rohde, LA.; Busnello, E.; Wolf, A.; Zomer, A.; Shansis, F.; Martins, S. and Tramontina, S., (1997). Maternity blues in Brazilian women. *Acta Psychiatrica Scandinavia*. Vol. 95, No. 3, pp. 231-235.

Sam, D., (2006a). Acculturation: Conceptual background and core components. In: *The handbook of acculturation psychology,* Sam, D. & Berry, IW. pp. 11-26. Cambridge University Press, Cambridge, UK

Sam, D., (2006b). Acculturation and health. In: *The handbook of acculturation psychology,* Sam, D. & Berry, IW. pp. 452-468. Cambridge University Press, Cambridge, UK

Savage, G., (1875). Observations on the insanity of pregnancy and childbirth. *Guy's Hospital Report*. Vol. 20, pp. 83-117.

Spielberger, CD.; Gorsuch, RL. and Lushene, RE., (1970). *Manual for the State-Trait Anxiety Inventory*. Consulting Psychologists Press, Palo Alto (Calif).

Skouteris, H.; Wertheim, EH.; Rallis, S.; Milgrom, J. and Paxton, SJ., (2009). Depression and anxiety through pregnancy and the early postpartum: an examination of prospective relationships. *Journal of Affective Disorders*. Vol. 13, No.3, pp. 303-308.

Stewart, DE.; Gagnon, A.; Saucier, JF.; Wahoush, O. and Dougherty, G., (2008). Postpartum depression symptoms in newcomers. *Canadian Journal of Psychiatry*. Vol. 53, No 2, pp. 121-124 .

Stuchbery, M.; Matthey, S. and Barnett, B., (1998). Postnatal depression and social supports in Vietnamese, Arabic and Anglo-Celtic mothers. *Social Psychiatry and Psychiatric Epidemiology*. Vol. 33, No. 10, pp. 483-490.

Taloyan, M.; Johansson, LM.; Johansson, SE.; Sundquist, J. and Koctürk, TO., (2006). Poor self-reported health and sleeping difficulties among Kurdish immigrant men in Sweden. *Transcultural Psychiatry*. Vol.43, No.3, pp. 445-461.

Taniguchi, H. and Baruffi, G., (2007). Childbirth overseas: the experience of Japanese women in Hawaii. Nursing and Health Sciences. Vol. 9, No. 2, pp. 90-95.

Tsukasaki, M.; Ohta, Y.; Oishi, K.; Miyaichi, K. and Kato, N., (1991). Types and characteristics of short-term course of depression after delivery: using Zung's Self Rating Depression Scale. *Japanese Journal of Psychiatry and Neurology*. Vol.45, No. 3, pp. 565-576.

Ugarizza, DN., (1992). Postpartum affective disorders: incidence and treatment. *Journal of Psychosocial Nursing and Mental Health Services*. Vol. 30, No. 5, pp. 29-32.

Yamashita, H.; Yoshida, K.; Nakano, H. and Tashiro, N., (2000). Postnatal depression in Japanese women. Detecting the early onset of postnatal depression by closely monitoring the postpartum mood. *Journal of Affective Disorders*. Vol. 58, pp. 145-154.

Yoshida, K.; Yamashita, H.; Ueda, M. and Tashiro, N., (2001). Postnatal depression in Japanese mothers and the reconsideration of 'Satogaeri bunben'. *Pediatrics International*. Vol.43, No. 2, pp. 189-93.

Yoshida, K.; Marks, MN.; Kibe, N.; Kumar, R.; Nakano, H. and Tashiro, N., (1997). Postnatal depression in Japanese women who have giver birth in England. *Journal of Affective Disorders*. Vol. 43, pp. 69-77.

Zelkowitz, P.; Saucier, JF.; Wang, T.; Katofsky, L.; Valenzuela, M. and Westreich, R., (2008). Stability and change in depressive symptoms from pregnancy to two months postpartum in childbearing immigrant women. *Archives of Women Mental Health*. Vol. 11, No. 1, pp. 1-11.

# 8

# Perinatal Depression in Minority and Underserved Rural Women

Guo Wei, Frankie D. Powell,
Veronica K. Freeman and Leonard D. Holmes
*University of North Carolina at Pembroke*
*USA*

## 1. Introduction

Perinatal depression among ethnic minority women is an understudied area of research. More specifically, prior to conducting interventions among this particular population, an extensive understanding of this knowledge base is necessary. Moreover, we are more aware of the multiple interrelationships between depression and various physical diseases, as well as socio-economic conditions and lifestyles. This chapter will explore that knowledge base and offer suggestions for future studies through an approach of social cognitive theory and the investigation of a well-mixed tri-racial and bi-ethnic sample.

## 2. Background

### 2.1 Definition of terms

Depression occurs across the population and throughout the life span. All women are at risk. The prevalence of perinatal depression is about the same as at other times in a woman's life (O'Hara, 1997). However, the consequences of perinatal depression are more compelling, as perinatal depression affects not only the women but their unborn babies, new babies, young children and the entire family support system.

The signs and symptoms of depression include depressed mood, tearfulness, sleep or appetite disturbances, nervousness or anxiety, irritability, weight gain or loss, loss of interest and pleasure, low energy, loss of concentration, guilt, hopelessness and thoughts of harming one's self or one's infant. Depressive symptoms may range from mild to severe. Severe symptoms often include thoughts of dying or suicide, wanting to flee or get away, being unable to feel love for the unborn baby or infant and having thoughts of hurting or not being able to protect the child.

Perinatal depression encompasses major and minor depressive episodes that occur either during pregnancy or within the first 12 months following delivery. Major depression is a distinct clinical syndrome for which treatment is clearly required (American Psychiatric Association, 2000), whereas the definition and management of minor depression are less clear.

### 2.2 Prevalence of perinatal depression

Global and national data indicate that depression in the general population has implications for both short-term (episodic) and long-term (chronic) mental health disability. Both can lead to traumatic outcomes for individuals and their families. For example, the World Health Organization (WHO) predicts that by 2020, depression will reach second place in the ranking of disability-adjusted life years (DALYs) calculated for all ages and both sexes. Within the context of the implications of depression as a major worldwide mental health disease, this chapter focuses on the critical impact of perinatal depression among minority and underserved rural women.

A national review by Gaynes et al. (Gaynes et al., 2005) on the prevalence of perinatal depression in the United States concluded that, for major and minor depression, the final combined estimates of point prevalence ranged between 8.5 percent and 11.0 percent at different times during pregnancy and between 6.5 percent and 12.9 percent at different times during the first year postpartum. Still, precise levels of the incidence of perinatal depression appear uncertain. Published estimates of the rates of major and minor depression in the postpartum period range widely—from 5 percent to more than 25 percent of new mothers, depending upon the assessment method, the timing of the assessment and population characteristics (O'Hara & Swain, 1996; Llewellyn, Stowe & Nemeroff, 1997; Yonkers et al., 2001).

Studies of prevalence included both white and African American women in samples. However, Native American and Hispanic women have not generally been included, thereby limiting the knowledge of perinatal depression in ethnic minority women. Only a few studies have begun to address this gap. In fact, as pointed out by Gaynes et al., "Prevalence studies need to provide better accountability of the racial and ethnic mix of perinatal depression in the U.S. population, as perinatal depression rates differ among various racial and ethnic groups. *The absence of information on nonwhite populations was dramatic,"* which comprises an interest of this chapter.

## 3. Conceptual framework

### 3.1 Definition of the concept

Defining depression is integral to the discussion of its impact on ethnic minority rural women. Depression is a biological, psychotic or psychosocial disorder often marked by depressed mood, nervousness or anxiety, inactivity, difficulty in thinking and concentration, emotional lability, tearfulness, sleep or appetite disturbance, weight gain or loss, loss of interest and pleasure, low energy, feelings of dejection, sadness and hopelessness, feelings of shame or loss of self, mental illness, feelings of guilt and suicidal tendencies. A history of depression and/or a family history of mood or anxiety disorders are significant risk factors for depression. Particularly during the perinatal period, a mother's desire to flee or get away, inability to feel love for the unborn baby or infant and thoughts of hurting or being unable to protect the infant are especially troubling.

Women bear the burden of responsibility associated with being wives, mothers and caregivers. In many underserved populations, women have considerable mental health needs; however, the conception of mental health in women has been limited as have attempts to protect and promote it. The weathering hypothesis (Geronimus, 1992) proposes that the health of African American and Native American women may begin to deteriorate in early adulthood as a physical consequence of cumulative socioeconomic disadvantage. African American and Native American women who are believed to be in poorer health than non-Hispanic white women, have a larger chance than non-Hispanic white women of experiencing poorer birth outcomes; however, they are also more sensitive than non-Hispanic white women to an intervention (such as an adequate perinatal care) that improves maternal health and birth outcomes. Hispanic women, whose health and birth outcomes are "better than expected," are receiving the lowest rates of perinatal care. When the health issues of women have been addressed in these populations, activities have tended to focus on issues associated with reproduction—such as family planning and bearing of children—while the mental health of women has been relatively neglected. Understanding perinatal depression in ethnic minority rural women requires a theoretical lens that helps explain how depression affects these women and their families. Social cognitive theory (SCT) is one such theory.

### 3.2 Application/relationship to postpartum depression

Social cognitive theory provides a framework for understanding, predicting and changing human behavior. The theory identifies human behavior as an interaction of personal factors, behavior and the environment (Bandura, 1977, 1986, 1989, 2001). In the model, the interaction between the person and behavior involves the influences of a person's thoughts and actions. The interaction between the person and the environment involves human beliefs and cognitive competencies that are developed and modified by social influences and structures within the environment. The third interaction, between the environment and behavior, involves a person's behavior determining the aspects of his or her environment, and in turn, their behavior is modified by that environment. In short, the three factors—environment, people and behavior—are constantly influencing one another. Behavior is not simply the result of the environment and the person, just as the environment is not simply the result of the person and behavior (Glanz et al., 2002). According to Jones (Jones, 1989), "the fact that behavior varies from situation to situation may not necessarily mean that behavior is controlled by situations but rather that the person is construing the situations differently and thus the same set of stimuli may provoke different responses from different people or from the same person at different times."

The application of this theory involves understanding the interrelationships between personal factors (in the form of cognitive, affective and biological events) and the external environment. Perinetal depression, for example, involves the knowledge a woman has about pregnancy and the clinical matters associated with it—how the woman feels about her pregnancy. It also involves the lived experience of the woman. Women who live in different environments see and respond to those environments through different lenses. Steven Covey has alluded to this concept when, in *The 7 Habits of Highly Effective People,* he states, "We must look at the lens through which we see the world, as well as the world we see, and that the lens itself shapes how we interpret the world." (Covey, 2004)

### 3.3 Specifically applied to ethnic minority women

According to the National Center for Law and Economic Justice (2010), African Americans, Native Americans and Hispanic Americans are more likely than others to live in poverty or deep poverty. This is especially true for racial and ethnic women who are the heads of their household and their families. Viewing, interpreting and responding to a highly impoverished environment might very well be a contributing factor to depression.

The depression status of some postpartum women may have become serious enough (e.g. major depression and minor depression), that treatment and/or intervention is required. On the other hand, for other postpartum women the level of depression is minimal, and these women can be treated by enrolling in education and training programs. A natural question arises: Why do some women experience major or minor depression while others do not? To answer this fundamental question, an appropriate method is to explore the differences between the two groups of women regarding their physical diseases, social factors, mental health aspects, personal behaviors and lifestyles among other environments. Such differences can be captured by using the social cognitive theory, which explains how people acquire and maintain certain behavioral patterns. SCT also provides the basis for intervention strategies (Bandura, 1997). The social cognitive theory is relevant to health communication. In fact, this theory deals with cognitive, emotional aspects and aspects of behavior for understanding behavioral change. The concepts advanced by this theory provide opportunities for new behavioral research in health education, ideas, insights, and understanding for other theoretical areas, such as psychology.

By employing the social cognitive theory and implementing its derived strategies, health professionals can better understand the relationships among pregnant women's personal factors, environment factors and behavior factors. As a result, this approach can greatly improve the access to perinatal women living in rural communities, thus increasing participation and retention in health programs. SCT is useful for establishing a basis on which to build a mutual trust between the health providers and perinatal women.

## 4. Overview of studies of postpartum depression: A review of the literature

A review of recent literature indicates the paucity of research about rural Native American and Hispanic women. This limited research underscores the need for data regarding these underserved populations. This review includes designs, methodology (including screening instruments and their reliability) and intervention and treatment models of perinatal depression. Our review includes publications on the studies of postpartum (and prenatal) depression in the past three decades.

Gaynes et al. concluded that up to 19.2 percent of new mothers may have either major or minor PPD in the first three months after giving birth (Gaynes et al., 2005). They also pointed out that, when discussing prevalence studies for PPD, it is clear that more quantitative research is needed to account for racial and ethnic differences. Longitudinal studies should be conducted to identify periods of peak prevalence over the first 12 months after birth. The limited number of published studies hampers the ability of clinicians to plan for the best times and places to screen and intervene. If the prevalence of this mood disorder peaks after six weeks, then screening programs need to be put into place in clinical settings other than obstetrics, such as family practice and pediatrics.

As such, depression in the general population has been extensively studied by many researchers in the past three decades (Beck, 2008). However, for postpartum depression, samples of those studies consisted of primarily white American and African American women, leaving the depressive status of other racial/ethnic groups, e.g., Native and Hispanic Americans, essentially unknown. A main purpose of our previous studies (Baker et al., 2005; Wei et al., 2008) and the present study is to eliminate or reduce such a knowledge gap.

### 4.1 Screening tools

The Edinburgh postnatal depression scale (EPDS) has been widely used in clinical settings to identify possible depressed women after giving birth. Peindl et al. (Peindl et al., 2004) investigated the effectiveness of the EPDS for major depression. The outcome of their study was identification of a recurrence of major depression in the first year postpartum by means of a clinical interview and use of the EPDS. Participants were pregnant women who had experienced a previous episode of postpartum-onset major depression (PPMD) but were well during their index pregnancy. This study was part of a double-blind, randomized clinical trial in which new mothers received nortriptyline or placebo within 24 hours following delivery for the prevention of PPMD. An earlier study regarding the development of the EPDS was given by Cox, Holden and Sagovsky (Cox, Holden & Sagovsky, 1987).

In additions to EPDS, other depression screening tools have been adopted. Recent research on the accuracy of alternative screening tools has been conducted for the Beck Depression Inventory II (BDI-II), and the Postpartum Depression Screening Scale (PDSS) (Chaudron et al., 2010). These approaches claim to identify major depressive disorder (MDD) or minor depressive disorder (MnDD) among low-income, urban mothers attending well-child care visits during their postpartum year. Large proportions of low-income, urban mothers attending WCC visits experienced MDD or MnDD during the postpartum year. In general, the EPDS, BDI-II, and PDSS are very useful in identifying depression, but scoring may need to be altered to identify depression more accurately among urban, low-income mothers.

For women with major depression alone, specificity for all screeners (the BDI, the PDSS and the EPDS) was relatively high and overlapped substantially. This finding suggests that a positive screen was accurate in identifying major depression; that is, the risk that a screen with one of these instruments would be falsely positive was low. By contrast, sensitivities varied much more. The EPDS and the PDSS appeared to be more sensitive (with estimates ranging from 0.75 to 1.0 at different thresholds) than the BDI instruments (with estimates from 0.32 to 0.68), but the wide confidence intervals overlapped nearly completely. Thus, the research findings were not supported, i.e., that the sensitivity estimates using the different tools were different (Gaynes et al., 2005).

### 4.2 Screening for risk factors

According to the American College of Obstetricians and Gynecologists Committee (ACOG Committee), psychosocial screening of all women seeking perinatal evaluation or care should be performed regardless of social status, educational level or race and ethnicity. Because problems may arise during perinatal period that were not present at the initial visit, it is best to perform psychosocial screening at least once in every three months to increase the likelihood of identifying important issues and reducing poor birth outcomes. Screening should include assessment of barriers to care, unstable housing, unintended pregnancy, communication barriers, nutrition, tobacco use, substance abuse, depression, safety, intimate partner violence and stress (ACOG Committee, 2006; Dobson & Dozois, 2008).

To clarify whether screening adults for depression in primary care settings improves recognition, treatment and clinical outcomes, Pignone et al. searched the Medline database for data from 1994 through August 2001. Other relevant articles were located through systematic searches of Medline from 1966 to 1994. Other data was taken from the Cochrane depression, anxiety, and neurosis database; hand searches of bibliographies; and extensive peer reviews. The researchers reviewed randomized trials conducted in primary care settings that examined the effect of screening for depression on identification, treatment or health outcomes, including trials that tested integrated, systematic support for treatment after identification of depression. Meta-analysis suggests that, screening and feedback reduced the risk for persistent depression (summary relative risk, 0.87 [95% CI, 0.79 to 0.95]). When combined with traditional care, screening for depression can improve outcomes, particularly when screening is coupled with system changes that help ensure adequate treatment and follow-up (Pignone et al., 2002).

### 4.3 Among minority and low-income women: Health disparities

Kozhimannil et al. (2001) investigated racial/ethnic differences in mental health care associated with postpartum depression in a multiethnic cohort of Medicaid recipients. The study included logistic regression for initiation of antidepressant medication or outpatient mental health visits within six months of delivery, follow-up and continued mental health care. There were significant racial/ethnic differences in depression-related mental health care after delivery. Suboptimal treatment was prevalent among all low-income women in the study. However, race- and ethnicity-based disparities in the initiation and continuation of postpartum depression care were particularly troubling and warrant clinical and policy attention. With analyses controlling for clinical factors, the odds of initiating treatment after delivery were significantly lower for African Americans and Hispanics compared with whites. Among those who initiated treatment, African Americans and Hispanics were less likely than whites to receive follow-up treatment or continued care. Among those who initiated antidepressant treatment, African American and Hispanic women were less likely than whites to refill a prescription. There were significant racial-ethnic differences in depression-related mental health care after delivery.

In contrast, for prenatal depression, research was conducted where risk factors for major prenatal depression among African American women were studied (Luke et al., 2009). They determined the prevalence and risk factors for major prenatal depression among low-income African American women, and used logistic regression to identify risk factors for major prenatal depression. The risk for major prenatal depression increases about five-fold among low-income African American women from age 30 as compared to teen mothers. The results are consistent with the weathering effect that results from years of cumulative stress burden due to socioeconomic marginalization and discrimination. Older African American mothers may benefit from routine prenatal depression screening for early diagnosis and intervention.

Plant and Sachs-Ericsson (Plant & Sachs-Ericsson, 2004) examined the depressive symptoms and prevalence of major depression among members of ethnic and racial minorities and white people from a large random sample. Minority group members experienced more depressive symptoms and a marginally higher prevalence of major depression than did white participants. These effects were mediated by participants' problems meeting their basic needs. Especially, minority group members reported more problems meeting their basic needs, and these problems were associated with an increased risk for depression and depressive symptoms. Interestingly, minority group members also reported a higher quality of interpersonal functioning than white participants did, which appeared to suppress the relationship between ethnicity and depression. However, measuring "interpersonal functioning" may be problematic.

Other quantitative work has explored the relationship between race and depression. Segre, O'Hara and Losch examined the extent to which race/ethnicity is a risk factor for depressed mood in late pregnancy and the early postpartum period, apart from its relationship with other demographic and infant outcome variables (Segre, O'Hara & Losch, 2006). Compared to white women, African American women were significantly more likely to report depressed mood (95% CI = 1.03 - 1.52); Hispanic women were significantly less likely to report being depressed (95% CI = 0.61 - 0.88). Moreover, authors also explored the role of social support in understanding the above findings.

Zayas, Jankowski and McKee (2005) studied parenting competency in a major life transition occurring within the context of an impoverished urban environment (Zayas, Jankowski & McKee, 2005). They also explored associations with depression, social support and life events. A sample of 182 African American and Hispanic mothers educated at community health centers in low-income urban areas completed measures early in the third trimester and again at three months postpartum. Across time, the levels of reported parental efficacy and satisfaction increased, while depressive symptoms decreased. Experiences at community health centers positively influenced women's experience of parenting satisfaction and feelings of efficacy before and after their babies were born.

Postpartum depression is prevalent in approximately 10 to 20% of women in the United States. Studies by Segre and colleagues, suggest that women of low income are at a higher risk of experiencing PPD than their more affluent counterparts, and African American women are more likely to suffer from PPD than both Hispanic and white women (Segre et al., 2006, 2007). Their first study focused on the income, education, marital status, number of children and occupational prestige of 4,332 women who, on average, gave birth 4.6 months prior to the research evaluation. These results indicate that social status is a significant predictor of PPD, with income as the strongest predictor. Their second study examined race and ethnicity as a factor for PPD. Data from the survey revealed that 15.7% of all women exhibited a single depressive item. African American women were most likely to report a depressive mood, while Hispanic women were least likely to report a depressive mood. Both studies emphasized the need for early PPD identification programs and strong social support for women with newborns.

### 4.4 Treatment and interventions

Appleby et al. (Appleby et al., 1997) studied the effectiveness of fluoxetine and cognitive - behavioral counseling. They used a randomized, controlled treatment trial, double-blind in relation to drug treatment, with four treatment cells: fluoxetine or placebo plus one or six postnatal sessions of counseling for a sample of 87 women at six to eight postnatal sessions. Seventy percent of the participants completed 12 weeks of treatment. The Edinburgh postnatal depression scale and the Hamilton depression scale were used. Highly significant improvement was seen in all four treatment groups. The improvement in subjects receiving fluoxetine was significantly greater than in those receiving placebo. The improvement after six sessions of counseling was significantly greater than after a single session. Interaction between counseling and fluoxetine was not statistically significant. These differences were evident after one week, and improvement in all groups was complete after four weeks. They concluded that both fluoxetine and cognitive-behavioral counseling given as a course of therapy are effective treatments for nonpsychotic depression in postnatal women. After an initial session of counseling, additional benefit results from either fluoxetine or further counseling but there seems to be no advantage to receiving both.

A pilot study was conducted to examine the initial acceptability, feasibility and effectiveness of the ROSE program (**R**esearch, **O**bservation, **S**ervice and **E**ducation) in the College of Medicine of the University of Cincinnati, using a brief, interpersonally based intervention in a group of low income, rural African American pregnant women at risk for PPD (Crockett et al., 2008). Participants were randomly assigned to the ROSE program or to treatment as usual (TAU). The women in the intervention condition reported significantly better postpartum adjustment at three months postpartum than women in the TAU group. Those in the ROSE program reported improvement in depressive symptoms over time, whereas women in the TAU group did not evidence such changes.

### 4.5 Relation to social supports

Surkan et al. examined the relationship of social support and social networks to symptoms of depression in a multiethnic sample of early postpartum women (Surkan et al., 2006). Univariate statistics assessed the relationship between Center for Epidemiologic Studies of Depression Scale (CES-D score) and each of the independent variables. Multivariate linear regression models included core socio-demographic variables alone, the core model with each of the social support and social network variables added separately, and all variables together. They evaluated interactions between race and social support, race and social networks and social support and social networks. As may be predicted, both social support and social networks were statistically significant and independently related to depressive symptomatology.

### 4.6 Recent findings

Knowledge regarding PPD remains incomplete at present. Despite the current classification of postpartum depression, doctors and clinicians with experience treating depressed mothers often note specific differences between unipolar depression and the depression that occurs immediately after childbirth. Silverman et al. (Silverman et al., 2011) recently used state-of-the-art brain imaging technology, functional magnetic resonance imaging (fMRI), to assess the neuroanatomical responsivity of the amygdala in women six to eight weeks postpartum and to understand how the brains of women with postpartum depression differ from non-depressed postpartum woman. While contemporary diagnostic nosology characterizes postpartum depression (PPD) as a specifier of a major depressive disorder (MDD), this traditional classification continues to be questioned. fMRI holds the promise of helping to characterize the neuroanatomical dysfunction associated with dysregulated emotion after childbirth. Postpartum depression (PPD) is nosologically classified as a specifier of a major depressive disorder (MDD); however specific differences in the clinical presentation of PPD have been identified (Cooper et al., 2007).

According to Silverman, depression comes in two types: unipolar and bipolar (see also, Verinder, 2010). Unipolar depression is characterized by severe depression, whereas bipolar type depressions include times of unusually elevated mood or energy—referred to as mania or hypomania. In the DSM-IV, the diagnostic manual used by psychiatrist and psychologists, postpartum depression is classified as a unipolar type depression. The results of the Silverman study suggest this classification might be inaccurate.

## 5. Overview of the methodologies used to study postpartum depression

### 5.1 Description of the setting

The purpose of this study was to examine the relationship between different levels of postpartum depression and the concomitant intervention. The setting of this study was the southeastern section of North Carolina, commonly known as the Sandhills, in Robeson County. Its population is very diverse (U.S. Census 2000): Lumbee Indian (46,896 or 38.0%; 1.2% for NC, 0.9% national), African American (30,973 or 25.1%; 21.6% for NC, 12.3% national), white (40,460 or 32.8%) and those of Hispanic origin (5,994 or 4.9%). The Hispanic population is rapidly growing, increased from 704 in 1990 to 5,994 in 2000 (850% increase). While the county population based on the 2010 census is not available yet, the predicated Hispanic population accounts for approximately 10 percent of the county population. In fact, for 2005 to 2007, Hispanic infants (an average of 385 births per year) accounted for 17.7 percent of all infants in the county (annual average live births 2,177 in 2005-2007). Two previous studies on postpartum depression (Baker et al., 2005; Wei et al., 2008) and a recent analysis of the depression during pregnancy (unpublished) have demonstrated extremely high rates of postpartum depression and prenatal depression in Robeson County.

### 5.2 Sample designs

Postpartum depression in white and African American women has been studied by many researchers (Beck, 1995, 2003; Amankwaa, 2003). The absence of information about other populations is striking (Gaynes et al., 2005). In particular, the depressive status of Native American and Hispanic women is essentially unknown; a direct comparison among African American, Hispanics, Native American, and white women remains a gap in the literature.

Our research addressed such a gap by using data obtained from Robeson County, North Carolina, through our Healthy Start Corps (HSC) project, which has been funded by the Health Resources and Services Administration (HRSA), the U.S. Department of Health and Human Services since 1998. Between September 1, 2002 and January 31, 2006, the HSC project and its clinical partner Robeson Healthcare Corporation (RHCC) recruited 1,245 postpartum clients from Robeson County, North Carolina, for treatment. It should be noted that the women administered Postpartum Depression Screening Scale (PDSS) were not randomly selected for two reasons: 1) the RHCC serves the primarily socio-economically underrepresented population in Robeson County; 2) the policies for this project require services be provided primarily to low income Native American and African American women. As a result, approximately 52% (645) of the 1,245 postpartum clients received the PDSS screenings at the six-weeks postpartum, with subsequent clinical referral as warranted. However, because of the timelines of reports, data analysis was conducted two times: 586 women (for disparities in PPD) and all the 645 women (for effectiveness of treatment and interventions on PPD), respectively.

The population studied is comprised of high-risk women who reflect the ethnic, social and cultural composition of Robeson County. The study group includes Healthy Start eligible women in Robeson County, North Carolina that initially visit the county health department and meet at least three of the following criteria for admission into Healthy Start: inadequate housing, relationship problems, adolescent mother, STD/HIV, poor pregnancy outcomes, spousal abuse/neglect, tobacco/alcohol/drug use or abuse, conflict/violence in the home, no perinatal care, missed appointment, illiteracy, financial problem, cultural/racial disparity, poor nutrition and/or history of depression.

The project's scope covered home-based preconceptional health through postpartum and interconceptional phases for high-risk mothers and infants. HSC cooperates with RHCC (2002 to 2006), Robeson County Health Department (since 2006) and other providers to deliver perinatal services for high-risk prenatal, postpartum and interconceptional women as well as infants. Perinatal health assessment, risk factors and depression screens aligned with continuous counseling and goal setting resulted in better birth outcomes, healthier behaviors, reduced risks and improved self-esteem of clients.

To achieve representative samples of participants, stratified and tree classification, and Bayesian methods were employed (Kadane, 1996). Table 1 summarizes the racial/ethnic distributions of the sample, along with comparisons to the racial/ethnic distributions of relevant populations (U.S. Census 2000). Native American and Hispanic women were oversampled; white women were undersampled.

| Group | Sample | | Robeson County (%) | North Carolina (%) | USA (%) |
|---|---|---|---|---|---|
| | No. | % | | | |
| Non-Hispanic Native | 305 | 52.00% | 37.7% (Lumbee Tribe) | 1.20% | 0.70% |
| Non-Hispanic African | 142 | 24.20% | 25.00% | 21.40% | 12.10% |
| Non-Hispanic White | 51 | 8.70% | 30.80% | 70.20% | 69.10% |
| Hispanic | 81 | 13.80% | 4.90% | 4.70% | 12.50% |
| Other* | 7 | 1.20% | 1.60% | 2.50% | 5.60% |
| Total | 586 | 100% | 100% | 100% | 100% |

* Non-Hispanic individuals of other races and non-Hispanic individuals of two or more races.

Table 1. Racial-ethnic distributions of the sample and population

The goal of this research was two-fold: 1) to estimate the prevalence of postpartum depression for African American, Hispanic, Native American, and white women and determine any presence of racial or ethnic differences and disparities; and 2) to integrate research findings and work in concert with the case management teams for the design of more targeted and feasible admission procedures and more effective intervention strategies and treatment plans. The first analysis included 586 of the 645 women, and the main purpose was to study racial/ethnic disparities (Wei et al., 2008). The second analysis included all the 645 women, and the main purpose was to investigate the effectiveness of the program interventions and treatment plans, based on the comparison of the initial screening results with follow-up screening results. The PDSS screenings were administered by the team supervisor, nurses, social workers, outreach workers and case managers trained in data collection and handling client confidential information.

### 5.3 Screening tool: Postpartum Depression Screening Scale (PDSS)

The PDSS is a self-report instrument with 35 items measuring depression and 10 for demographic characteristics. The 35 items are also grouped into seven symptom subscales: sleeping or eating disturbances, anxiety/insecurity, emotional lability, mental confusion, loss of self, guilt/shame and suicidal thoughts. If the score for the first seven items (short score) is less than 14, a full screening is not administered, and the client is classified as Normal Adjustment. If a score of 14 or higher is identified, the client completes the remaining 28 items in the same day. If the full score is between 60 and 79, the client is classified as Minor Depression; if 80 or higher, the client is classified as Major Depression. In either case, the client is referred for appropriate intervention or treatment.

### 5.4 Data analysis methods and software tools

To explore risk factors of depression, the factor analysis method was first used to extract the characteristics of these women. The assumptions required include no outlier, adequate sample size, linearity, no perfect multicollinearity and linear data. Factor analysis is a statistical method by which the regularity and order in phenomena can be discerned. It is a detection method for data structure, but it is different from principal component analysis whose purpose is data deduction (Hair et al., 1992; Dillon & Goldstein, 1984). Factor analysis is used to investigate interdependencies between variables in an effort to explore a new set of variables (fewer in number than the original set of variables), which express commonality among the original variables. The essence of factor analysis is to simplify complex and diverse relationships that exist among the set of observed variables by uncovering common dimensions or factors that link together the seemingly unrelated variables. Another method used was the structural equation models approach that allows both confirmatory and exploratory modeling and is suited to both theory testing and theory development.

Four different approaches for assessing reliability analysis were considered for the reliability of the instruments measuring the tri-racial and bi-ethnic population: test-retest reliability, internal consistency reliability, split half reliability and inter-rater reliability. Confidence intervals of the rates of major and minor depression by group were estimated (Table 2), followed by statistical tests to first determine the differences among these rates and then explore the differences in variations of full scores and differences in mean full scores between groups. Risk assessment was performed with factor analysis and correlation methods (Wei et al., 2008).

| Racial or Ethnic Group | PDSS Short Scale (Total score of first seven items) | | | | | PDSS Full Scale (Total score of all thirty five items) | | | | | | | | |
|---|---|---|---|---|---|---|---|---|---|---|---|---|---|---|
| | | | | | | | Major Depression (% in all 586 women) | | | | Minor Depression (% in all 586 women) | | | |
| | No | ≥ 14 | % | Lower 95% CI | Upper 95% CI | No | ≥ 80 | % | Lower 95% CI | Upper 95% CI | 60-79 | % | Lower 95% CI | Upper 95% CI |
| White | 51 | 23 | 45.1 | 31.4 | 58.8 | 24 | 9 | 17.6 | 7.2 | 28.1 | 10 | 19.6 | 8.7 | 30.5 |
| African | 142 | 47 | 33.1 | 25.4 | 40.8 | 48 | 21 | 14.8 | 9.0 | 20.6 | 14 | 9.9 | 5.0 | 14.8 |
| Native | 305 | 126 | 41.3 | 35.8 | 46.8 | 128 | 57 | 18.7 | 14.3 | 23.1 | 32 | 10.5 | 7.1 | 13.9 |
| Hispanic[1] | 81 | 5 | 6.2 | 0.95 | 11.5 | 4 | 2 | 2.5 | -0.9 | 5.9 | 0 | 0.0 | 0.0 | 0.0 |
| Other | 6 | 2 | 33.3 | -4.4 | 71 | 4 | 1 | 16.7 | -13.1 | 46.5 | 1 | 16.7 | -13.1 | 46.5 |
| Total | 586 | 203 | 34.6 | 30.7 | 38.5 | 209 | 90 | 15.4 | 12.5 | 18.3 | 58 | 9.9 | 7.5 | 12.3 |

[1] Hispanic women are not included in the racial groups.

Table 2. Racial and Ethnic Prevalence of Postpartum Depression

The major factors (and their components - original 35 factors in the PDSS holding loadings larger than 0.70; factor loadings less than 0.40 dropped; standard regression coefficients used) were identified according to the order of significance where italic (component) factors had average ratings of "agree" or "strongly agree" from the 90 likely major depressive participants. The Henry Kaiser's eigenvalue-based rule (Rule of Thumb) was used: The total number of factors is chosen as the number of eigenvalues of the correlation matrix that are larger than one (Morrison, 1990). The software tools used included SAS and SPSS. The significant first seven items are:

1. Mental confusion (moving or pacing, *anxiety*, difficulty focusing on task, hard to make decisions, *anger, crazy, irritable*),
2. Suicidal thoughts (better off dead, seemed death, want to hurt self, want to leave the world, not normal),
3. Trouble sleeping and imaginary feeling (feeling not real, trouble sleeping, stranger to self, *hard back sleep, tossed and turned to sleep*, jump out of skin, *feel alone*),
4. Guilt or shame (not loving baby, felt baby better without me, felt failure as mother, hide thinking and feeling, not mother wanted to be, felt others better),
5. Loss of self (felt never be normal, *lost mind*, never happy),
6. Emotional lability (*overwhelmed, roller emotion*) and
7. Eating disturbance (should but not eat, lost appetite).

### 5.5 Racial differences and ethnic disparities (586 women)

Three racial groups (African American, Native and white) shared similar depression status. Major dissimilarities existed between the Hispanic group and the non-Hispanic group (Wei et al., 2008). The prevalence of depression at six weeks postpartum in a rural triracial population using the Beck and Gable PDSS found that Native American women had the highest rate of major depression (18.7%) and average rates of minor depression (10.5%). Although white women had the second highest rate of major depression (17.6%) and the highest rate of minor depression (19.6%), their average full score (76.1) was still significantly lower than that of Native American women (82.9) (at $\alpha = 0.23$) and slightly lower than that of African American women (78.9, major depression 14.8%). Hispanic women had the lowest rates of major and minor depression (2.5%) (Table 2).

## 6. Early intervention study - identification, intervention and treatment

This data supports the hypothesis that timing and quality of perinatal care received by the mother during pregnancy and in the postpartum period are critically important to both the mother and the infant. Early comprehensive perinatal care can promote improved perinatal health by providing health behavior advice, monitoring, early detection and treatment of risk factors and symptoms.

### 6.1 Screening with clinical setting

Healthy Start Corps (HSC) operates on the principle that prenatal counseling or early postpartum screening for depressive symptoms with subsequent intervention will lead to improved health outcomes for the mother and her infant. The postpartum clients in the program were all given at least one initial depression screening at six weeks postpartum, with possible screening results ranging within normal adjustment, significant symptoms of (minor) postpartum depression, or major postpartum depression. Women identified as at-risk for major and minor depression were given subsequent screenings in the fourth month and twelfth month after delivery. Literature on postpartum depression was distributed to all participants. All participants were provided one-on-one counseling and education regarding the differences between baby blues, postpartum depression and postpartum psychosis, signs and symptoms of depression, high risk factors for postpartum depression and the significance of public health concerns of postpartum depression.

As a participant of HSC, weekly home visits occurred until the client exhibited a stable mental and emotional status. Follow-up was made regarding mental health appointments and medication regimen effectiveness. Increased rest and support from family and friends were encouraged for childcare and chores in promoting optimal mental and emotional well-being. Participants were encouraged to engage in activities to promote increased socialization among other participants who had experienced many of the same postpartum depression episodes through group activities arranged by the HSC.

Because of religions, beliefs, traditions, lifestyles and desire for privacy and other reasons, it is a challenge for health professionals to access local communities and organizations and recruit program participants. This effort is especially difficult when recruiting for community-based programs, such as the U.S. National Healthy Start programs, which has been funded by the Health Resources and Services Administration of the U.S. Department of Health and Human Services since 1991. These programs focus on reducing infant mortality and eliminating health disparities by promoting adequate perinatal care for minority and underserved women. Efficient and experienced case managers could be placed into embarrassing situations when delivering home-based perinatal services, e.g. depression screens, as experienced by Healthy Start's interconceptional case management programs.

### 6.2 Interventions

Interventions Used for Normal Postpartum Participants (PDSS Short Score ≤ 13 or Full Score ≤ 59): Soon after giving birth (during the postnatal period), most new mothers experience mood swings and mild depression (baby blues). This condition usually peaks from a few days day after delivery to the end of the second week. Afterwards (during the postpartum period), for a majority of women, their bodies enter a normal adjustment category in response to changing postpartum hormone levels. One method of active prevention that was helpful for the HSC postpartum women was a brief intervention, derived from the principles of social learning theory and empirically validated as an effective methodology. These participants received the HSC- distributed literature on postpartum depression, were recommended to attend the HSC health education classes, were encouraged to get plenty of rest and elicit the support of family and friends for childcare and chores and were offered Healthy Start and Child Service Coordination as an additional source of support.

Methods of Treatment Used for Participants with Significant Symptoms of (Minor) Postpartum Depression (PDSS Full Score 60-79): One-on-one counseling was often provided by an HSC-trained social worker within the home for each woman, and a referral to a mental health agency was offered. These participants were educated on postpartum depression and were given additional literature on postpartum depression, including emergency contact numbers. These participants were also offered HSC health education classes and Child Service Coordination. A home visit was made weekly up until the eighth week postpartum for each woman by the maternity care coordinator (MCC) in order to evaluate her emotional status as well as the interaction with her infant. Again substantial rest and the support of family and friends for child care and chores were encouraged for optimal emotional well being. Screening occurred at varying times since postpartum mood disorders could be expressed in a variety of ways and at different time intervals. The HSC postpartum and interconceptional case management teams continued to use the PDSS tool to monitor all postpartum and interconceptional clients. All clients are provided one-on-one counseling on the differences between baby blues and postpartum depression/psychosis, the signs and symptoms of depression, high risk factors for postpartum depression, the public health concerns of postpartum depression and the role and approaches in providing information to the community on the signs and symptoms of postpartum depression.

Methods of Treatment Used for Participants with Major Postpartum Depression (PDSS Full Score ≥ 80): If depressive and psychiatric symptoms were first encountered within the clinical setting and a major postpartum depression screening was identified, a same day referral to a clinical physician was made. Further referrals were then made with an outside provider if psychiatric counseling was required, dependent upon the severity of conditions. Additionally counseling sessions were arranged by HSC with a local provider for up to four visits with costs being absorbed by HSC. Follow-up by HSC was carried out by verifying that participants kept appointments with the care provider and by rescheduling referral appointments as needed. Participants who had scores indicative of major depression were encouraged not to leave the facility without seeing a medical provider (MD, PA, or NP). The medical provider proceeded in extensive education with the participant regarding the postpartum depression screening results and encouraged the acceptance of a referral to a mental health professional. Antidepressant medications were usually prescribed by the medical provider. If there was concern regarding suicidal ideation or a threat of potential harm to others, the participant was referred for emergency services and immediate evaluation. Consent was sought for confiding in the spouse or significant others for education on the dangers of untreated major postpartum depression and intervention options. Again literature was given to the couple including emergency contact phone numbers (hospital, mental health agency, etc). HSC referrals and Child Service Coordination services were offered as well. The maternal care coordinator contacted the high-risk participant every other day for several days and made a home visit weekly up until eight weeks postpartum.

### 6.3 Initial screening results

The initial screening was administered at the sixth week postpartum to all the 645 women. Women in the whole sample showed similarities and dissimilarities by racial/ethnic group. These group averages are close for age, history of depression, treatment history, gravida, number of children, delivery method and low family income. Major differences included that Hispanic women had a lower education level than non-Hispanic women, but the highest breast feeding rate; white women had the highest percentage of marriages, while African American women had the lowest marriage percentage.

| | PDSS Short Scale | | | PDSS Full Scale | | | | |
|---|---|---|---|---|---|---|---|---|
| | Significant Symptoms | | | | Major Depression (% in all 645 women) | | Minor Depression (% in all 645 women) | |
| Race | No. | ≥ 14 | % | No. | ≥ 80 | % | 60-79 | % |
| White | 55 | 25 | 45.5 | 26 | 10 | 18.2 | 11 | 20 |
| African American | 157 | 49 | 31.2 | 50 | 21 | 13.4 | 16 | 10.2 |
| Native | 338 | 138 | 40.8 | 139 | 62 | 18.3 | 34 | 10.1 |
| Hispanic | 87 | 6 | 6.9 | 5 | 2 | 2.3 | 1 | 1.1 |
| Other | 8 | 3 | 37.5 | 5 | 1 | 12.5 | 2 | 25 |
| Total | 645 | 221 | 34.3 | 225 | 96 | 14.9 | 64 | 9.9 |

Table 3. Racial and Ethnic Disparities - Initial Screening

Table 3 summarizes the racial and ethnic disparities based on the PDSS short scale for the 645 women and the PDSS full scale for the 225 women who were required to take the full screen. The full scale screening determined 96 had major postpartum depression, and 64 had significant symptoms (minor depression). Note the percentages in all the tables are calculated on the basis of the original sample (645 postpartum women). The first column from left under PDSS full scale indicates the numbers of women who completed the full scale screening in relevant categories, respectively. With direct calculations from Table 3, the incidence of major and minor postpartum depression in the 645 women was (96+64)/645 = 24.8 percent. The results support previous racial data: Native women had the highest incidence of major postpartum depression (18.3%), followed by white women

(18.2%), African American women (13.4%), and finally Hispanic women (2.0%). White women were most likely to have minor postpartum depression (20.0%), followed by African American women (10.2%), Native American women (10.1) and finally Hispanic women (1.1%).

### 6.4 Depressive status of the postpartum women (follow-up screenings after intervention and treatment)

The follow-up PDSS full screening was conducted at the end of the fourth month after delivery for all women whose PDSS scores at the six-week postpartum were higher or equal to 60 (major or minor depression). Table 4 below shows the results, compared to Table 3 of the initial screening. This indicates a significant improvement for all racial/ethnic groups. Of the 160 (96+64) women who had major and minor depression (Table 3), 137 received the second screening (Table 4). For all women, the rate of major depression was reduced from 14.9% at six weeks postpartum to 3.7% (white: 18.2% to 1.8%; African American: 13.4% to 3.8%; Native American: 18.3% to 4.7%; Hispanic descent: 2.3% to 1.1%). For all women, the rate of minor depression dropped from 9.9 percent at six weeks postpartum to 4.0% (white: 20.0% to 5.5%; African American: 10.2% to 4.5%; Native American: 10.1% to 4.4%; Hispanic descent: 1.1% to 0.0%). The combined major and minor depression rate was reduced from 24.8% at six weeks postpartum, which is high compared to various estimates in other populations (Gaynes et al., 2005), to a level of 7.7%, which is close to the midrange of other populations. Hence, the outcomes from the interventions and treatments were significant. (If the sample size was larger, participants could be divided into a treatment group and a control group to admit a direct comparison.)

| | PDSS Short Scale | | | PDSS Full Scale | | | | |
|---|---|---|---|---|---|---|---|---|
| | Significant Symptoms | | | | Major Depression (% in all 645 women) | | Minor Depression (% in all 645 women) | |
| **Race** | No. | | | No. | $\geq$ 80 | % | 60-79 | % |
| White | 55 | | | 18 | 1 | 1.8 | 3 | 5.5 |
| African American | 157 | | | 31 | 6 | 3.8 | 7 | 4.5 |
| Native | 338 | | | 86 | 16 | 4.7 | 15 | 4.4 |
| Hispanic | 87 | | | 1 | 1 | 1.1 | 0 | 0 |
| Other | 8 | | | 1 | 0 | 0 | 1 | 12.5 |
| Total | 645 | | | 137 | 24 | 3.7 | 26 | 4 |

Note: Percentages are calculated using the basis of all 645 women to allow a comparison with Table 3.

Table 4. Improved Outcomes - Second PDSS Full Screening

Since 2006 the Healthy Start Corps program has added several supplemental questions to the PDSS regarding participants' demographic information, such as family income, employment status, education level and maternal smoking, and a total of 456 postpartum women were administered the PDSS and the supplemental questions. Of these participants, 161 smoked during postpartum period, 284 did not smoke, and 11 had an unknown status. Thirty-seven (23%) of the smokers received scores larger than or equal to 80 (major depression), and only 25 (8.8%) received scores larger than or equal to 80. Levels of depression are also associated with employment status and family income; 5.8% of full-time workers received a score 80 or higher, while 12.1% of part-time workers scored 80 or higher, and 15.2% of unemployed participants received a score 80 or higher. Moreover, the project also screened for prenatal depression since 2006.

## 7. Discussion and conclusions

Postpartum depression (PPD) is an issue critical to the health of women and their infants, as depressive episodes can become chronic or recurrent and lead to substantial impairments in the ability of an individual to handle daily responsibilities. In addition to the seriousness for the postpartum women, it is known that the period immediately following birth is a critical time for the newborn's development; postpartum depression can constitute a serious threat to the infant's well-being.

Major perinatal depression is considerably underdiagnosed, and many women with such symptoms live untreated. Therefore, mothers and their family members may suffer serious adverse effects, that could impact the emotional and psychological development of the child. A simple screening instrument like the PDSS, the PDIS, the BDI or BDI II (Gaynes et al., 2005) can increase the detection of major depression.

### 7.1 Cultural sensitivity and linguistic needs

Many barriers exist in raising awareness of and intervention of perinatal depression, including stigmatism, denial, transportation, childcare, access to care and, in some cases, lack of insurance when Medicaid is not an option. Health programs may strive to address these barriers in serving high-risk women by forming linkages with community providers and organizations that provide wide services and enrichment activities.

In addition to improving the delivery of treatment and intervention, providers of health programs must reduce cultural and linguistic barriers to perinatal services and support in rural and population-diverse communities. To achieve this goal, health programs and care providers should direct attention to cultural awareness, languages, easy-to-read materials, knowledge and skills, promotion of cultural and linguistic competence, attitudes, legally binding documents, and policies to enable effective cross-cultural working relationships. Family-driven and community-based outreach, flexible appointment times, home visits, and use of cultural brokers and traditional healers are possible approaches. Research and action staff must receive appropriate training to help assess clients' social, emotional and behavioral disorders or mental illness.

Native women are more likely to have inadequate health care, poor nutrition, high adolescent pregnancy rates, high incidences of living in sub-standard housing and, by far, the highest percentage of smoking tobacco during pregnancy. African Americans experience infant mortality and low birth weight rates double that of whites and suffer from nearly all major health causes because they often receive less and poorer quality health care. Hispanic women are generally in poorer health, although some of their health indicators are "better than expected," e.g., perinatal depression (known as an epidemiological paradox or the Hispanic paradox), or comparable to that of non-Hispanic white (i.e., infant mortality and low birthweight rates). Hispanic women have been found to initiate childbearing earlier and more likely to give birth to four or more children. Hispanic mothers continue to have children later in life than other women and receive inadequate health care.

### 7.2 Challenges - access to care and cultural influences

In 2010 a focus group study was conducted aimed at uncovering the reasons behind women's refusals and dropouts of various federal, state and community health programs. The focus group interviews and qualitative analysis uncovered several new concepts that contribute to health disparities. Several of the concepts relate directly to cultural and social practices common in Robeson County as well as other factors and barriers. Others relate to issues of trust and poverty. These concepts and the grounded theory method together can provide a basis for instrument developments in future (e.g., survey questionnaires) that can be implemented for the detection of refusals and dropouts from heath programs. Qualitative and quantitative analyses of focus group data and Healthy Start Corps data indicated that issues of trust play a role in healthcare. Subjects do not believe: 1) doctors have their best interests at heart, 2) doctors have up-to-date skill sets or equipment, 3) they will receive adequate care in the hospital or emergency room, and 4) medical personnel will not use race and class as a factor in determining treatments.

Most subjects commented on the role their culture plays in their diets, with many suggesting that a southern diet is filled with fried foods and sugar. One subject phrased it as, "We southerners like a little tea with our sugar and fried chicken." Some claimed that it was a combination of the southern culture and the Native American and African American poverty that led to "eating what you had." Several Native Americans said that their "typical diet" growing up was a breakfast of lard biscuits dipped into a mixture of bacon grease and sugar, a lunch of fatback and vegetables and a dinner of fatback or other cuts of pork and vegetables.

Cost of medical care is a great concern to all subjects regardless of employment and insurance status. Many of the subjects have been unemployed for several years; many have been without insurance for as many as 10 years. One pregnant woman who does have insurance claimed she skips appointments because she cannot afford the co-pays. Focus group participants also talked about alternative strategies, such as borrowing medicines from others who are insured or on Medicaid, using extra medicine around the house, going to the horse feed store or veterinarian to buy animal medicine to treat themselves and home remedies (some scientifically based; others mostly superstition).

### 7.3 Advantages and limitations of the study

The sample is a well-mixed tri-racial and bi-ethnic one, including Native Americans and Hispanic Americans. Using social cognitive theory in the study of depression opens a new door for examining perinatal and mental health. The classification of postpartum women into three categories according to severity of depression is an effective way to deliver appropriate and timely interventions and treatments. Moreover statistical methods, including risk factor analysis, are also a significant part of the study.

Limitations of this research include: 1) lack of information about diagnosed major and minor postpartum depression (thus a comparison between the PDSS screening results and actual depression cannot be compared), 2) lack of additional participant health risk information such as prenatal health and substance use and 3) although the original sample size for Hispanic women was not small, the number of Hispanic women who were required to complete PDSS full screening was inadequate.

### 7.4 Conclusions

Fundamental principles of human development attest to three interrelated processes that continue throughout the lifespan on an individual: biological and physical development and health; cognitive development; and socio-emotional development (Santrock, 2008). In addition, the individual is influenced by the social context of these developmental processes. Perinatal depression is both an expression of the link between and the interaction of these three processes within the context of the particular environment. Thus, it is impossible to extricate the findings of this study from the context in which the clients lived. The context included, but was not limited to, conditions of economic underdevelopment and comorbid health conditions, e.g., substance abuse, physical and sexual abuse, diabetes and obesity.

It is within the particular context of these ethnic minority rural women that early identification of postpartum depressive women with subsequent intervention and treatment was found to improve outcomes. The combined rate of major and minor depression was reduced from 24.8% (at six weeks postpartum), which is high compared to various estimates in literature for other populations (Gaynes et al., 2005; Cox & Murray, 1993; O'Hara & Swain, 1996; Llewellyn, Stowe & Nemeroff, 1997; Yonker et al., 2001), to a level of 7.7% (in the fourth month after delivery), which is close to the midrange of other populations. The classification of participants into the three categories based on their PDSS scores makes it possible to provide interventions and treatments at the appropriate levels.

Appropriate depression screening can improve health outcomes when combined with a system for treatment. Screening is an effective and feasible strategy in timely identification of depressive women. The Beck and Gable PDSS provided a clinically useful and cost-effective (compared with the clinical diagnosing process) screening instrument for early identification of depressive episodes. Depression is treatable and may not be resolved without treatment. Early identification and treatment by primary care clinicians or mental health specialists are essential.

### 7.5 Future research

Refusal of or dropping out of perinatal health services, including critical depression and other risk screen programs, are not uncommon, and these issues are more serious for some racial/ethnic groups (e.g., non-Hispanic African Americans and Native Americans). High refusal and dropout rates of underserved and minority women demonstrate the existence of significant gaps between services offered by the current perinatal care system and suitable perinatal care according to the perinatal women themselves. Perinatal women are not likely to accept an offer that does not fit their health needs, judged by their own point of view. To resolve this controversial situation, perinatal care plans and other interventions need to be "redesigned" by incorporating perinatal women's health needs and their view toward health programs. To understand their view, it is clearly necessary for health professionals to study the three factors—personal issues, environmental considerations, and behavioral aspects—of the women.

The social cognitive theory explains how people acquire and maintain certain behavioral patterns, while also providing the basis for intervention strategies (Bandura, 1997). Here, the "patterns" and "basis" as well as the relationships among the above three factors are critically useful information for designing and implementing more effective health programs. According to Levinson, the transition from late adolescence to early adulthood is characterized by the establishment of independence from parents, the exploration of establishing an adult identity, and the formation of life goals (Levinson, 1996). Thus, it is understandable that both the pregnancy and the context of the pregnancy influence the expectant mothers' view of independence, identity, and long-term goals. Her multi-layered socio-cognitive and socio-emotional response is inextricably linked to her depression or her lack of depression. Therefore, further study and wider utilization of this theory and the principles of human development are important, practical, and useful topics for future studies of perinatal depression. Moreover, the inclusion of studies that examine perinatal women's health through an exploration of the female reproductive life cycle from an evolutionary perspective may also be helpful in understanding this topic (Trevathan, 2010). Ultimately, we believe that a decrease in perinatal depression will occur through the elimination of perinatal risk factors, changing of risky behaviors and lifestyles, promotion of cultural and linguistic competence, and the reduction of racial/ethnic disparities.

## 8. Acknowledgments

This work was approved and supported by The University of North Carolina at Pembroke and the Healthy Start Corps project "Eliminating Disparities in Perinatal Health." The Healthy Start Corps project has been funded by the Maternal and Child Health Bureau, Health Resources and Services Administration, U.S. Department of Health and Human Services (Grant Number: H49MC00068) since 1998. This work is also supported by the Sartorius-Stedim Biotechnology Research Laboratory at The University of North Carolina at Pembroke, through an Extramural Associates Research Development Award (EARDA) from the National Institute of Child Health and Human Development (NICHD). Perinatal data analyzed in this work was from the Healthy Start Corps project's database. The annotated bibliography was well-achieved through the efforts of Mr. Dingyang Wei, who is currently a student in the Department of Mathematics at The University of North Carolina at Chapel Hill.

## 9. References

Amankwaa, L. C. (2003). Postpartum Depression among African-American Women. *Issues Ment Nurs*, Vol. 24, No. 3, (April-May 2003), pp. 297–316, ISSN 0161-2840

American College of Obstetricinas and Gynecologists (ACOG). (2006). Committee Opinion No. 343: Psychosocial Risk Factors: Perinatal Screening and Intervention. *Obstet Gynecol*, Vol. 108, No. 2, (August 2006), pp. 469-77, ISSN 0029-7844

American Psychiatric Association (APA). (2000). Practice Guideline for the Treatment of Patients with Major Depression (revision). *Am J Psychiatry*, Vol. 157, No. 4 Suppl, (April 2000), pp. 1-45, ISSN 0002-953X

Appleby, L., Warner, R., Whitton, A. & Faragher, B. (1997). A Controlled Study of Fluoxetine and Cognitive-behavioural Counselling in the Treatment of Postnatal Depression. *BMJ*, Vol. 314, No. 7085, (March 1997), pp. 932-936, ISSN 2044-6055

Baker, L., Cross, S., Greaver, L., Wei, G. & Lewis, R. (2005). Prevalence of Postpartum Depression in a Native American Population. *Matern & Child Health J*, Vol. 9, No. 1, (March 2005), pp 21-25, ISSN 1092-7875

Bandura, A. (1977). *Social Learning Theory*. Prentice-Hall, ISBN 978-013-8167-44-8, Englewood Cliffs, NJ, USA

Bandura, A. (1986). *Social Foundations of Thought and Action: A Social Cognitive Theory*. Prentice-Hall, ISBN 978-013-8156-14-5, Englewood Cliffs, NJ, USA

Bandura, A. (1989). Human Agency in Social Cognitive Theory. *Amer. Psychologist*, Vol. 44, No. 9, (September 1989), pp. 1175-1184, ISSN 0003-066X

Bandura, A. (1997). *Self-efficacy: The Exercise of Control*, W.H. Freeman, ISBN 978-071-6726-26-5, New York, NY, USA

Bandura, A. (2001). Social Cognitive Theory: An Agentic Perspective. *Annual Review of Psychology*, Vol. 52, No. 1, (February 2001), pp. 1-26, ISSN 0066-4308

Beck, C. T. (1995). The Effects of Postpartum Depression on Maternal-infant Interaction. *Nurs Res*, Vol. 44, No. 5, (September-October 1995), pp. 298–304, ISSN 0029-6562

Beck, C.T. & Gable R.K. (2002). *Postpartum Depression Screening Scale*, Western Psychological Services, Los Angeles, CA, USA

Beck, C. T. (2003). Recognizing and Screening for Postpartum Depression in Mothers of NICU Infants. *Adv Neonatal Care*, Vol. 3, No. 1, (February 2003), pp. 37–46, ISSN 1536-0903

Beck, C. (2008). State of the Science on Postpartum Depression (Parts 1 and 2). *MCN: The Amer. J. of Matern & Child Nurs*, Vol. 33, No. 2 & 3, (March-April 2008 & May-June 2008), pp. 121-126, 151-156, ISSN 0361-929X

Chaudron, L.H., Szilagyi, P.G., Tang, W., Anson, E., Talbot, N.L., Wadkins, H.I. & et al. (2010). Accuracy of Depression Screening Tools for Identifying Postpartum Depression among Urban Mothers. *Pediatrics*, Vol. 125, No. 3, (March 2010), pp. 609-617, ISSN 0031-4005

Cooper, C., Jones, L., Dunn, E., Forty, L., Haque, S. & Oyebode, F. & et al. (2007). Clinical Presentation of Postnatal and Non-postnatal Depressive Episodes. *Psychol Med*, Vol. 37, No. 9, (September 2007), pp. 1273–1280, ISSN 0033-2917

Covey, S. R. (2004). *The Seven Habits of Highly Effective People*, Free Press, ISBN 978-074-3269-51-3, New York, NY, USA

Cox, J.L., Holden, J.M. & Sagovsky, R. (1987). Detection of Postnatal Depression. Development of the 10-item Edinburgh Postnatal Depression Scale. *Br J Psychiatry*, Vol. 150, (June 1987), pp. 782-786, ISSN 0007-1250

Cox, J. L., Murray, D. & Chapman, G. (1993). A Controlled Study of the Onset, Duration and Prevalence of Postnatal Depression. *Br J Psychiatry,* Vol. 163, No. 1, (July 1993), pp. 27-31, ISSN 0007-1250

Crockett, K., Zlotnick, C., Davis, M., Payne, N. & Washington, R. (2008). A Depression Preventive Intervention for Rural Low-income African-American Pregnant Women at Risk for Postpartum Depression. *Archives of Women's Mental Health,* Vol. 11, No. 5-6, (December 2008) pp. 319-325, ISSN 1434-1816

Dillon, W. R. & Goldstein M. (1984). *Multivariate Analysis,* John Wiley & Sons, ISBN 978-047-1083-17-7, New York, NY, USA

Dobson, K.S. & Dozois, D. J. (2008). *Risk Factors in Depression,* Elsevier Science, ISBN 978-008-0450-78-0, Amsterdam, Netherlands

Gaynes, B.N., Gavin, N., Meltzer-Brody, S., Lohr, K.N., Swinson, T., Gartlehner, G., Brody, S. & Miller W.C. (2005). *Perinatal Depression: Prevalence, Screening Accuracy, and Screening Outcomes,* Rockville, MD, USA: RTI – International-University of North Carolina Evidence-based Practice Center, Report/Technology Assessment No. 119, Contract No. 290-02-0016

Geronimus, A.T. (1992). The Weathering Hypothesis and the Health of African-American Women and Infants: Evidence and Speculations, *Ethn. Dis.,* Vol. 2, No. 3, (Summer 1992), pp. 207-221, ISSN 1049-510X

Glanz, K., Rimer, B.K. & Lewis, F.M. (2002). *Health Behavior and Health Education. Theory, Research and Practice,* Wiley & Sons, ISBN 978-078-7957-15-5, San Francisco, CA, USA

Hair, J.F., Anderson, R., Tatham R. & Black, W.C. (1992). *Multivariate Data Analysis,* 3rd ed, Macmillan, ISBN 978-002-9465-64-6, New York, NY, USA

Jones, J. W. (1989). Personality and Epistemology: Cognitive Social Learning Theory as a Philosophy of Science, *Zygon's J of religion & Science,* Vol. 24, No. 1, (March 1989), pp. 23-38, ISSN 0591-2385

Kadane J.B. (1996). *Bayesian Methods and Ethics in a Clinical Trial Design,* John Wiley & Sons, ISBN 978-047-1846-80-2, New York, NY, USA

Kozhimannil, K.B., Trinacty, C.M., Busch, A.B., Huskamp, H.A. & Adams, A.S. (2011). Racial and Ethnic Disparities in Postpartum Depression Care among Low-income Women, *Psychiatric Services,* Vol. 62, (June 2011), pp. 619-625, ISSN 1075-2730

Lancaster, C.A., Gold, K.J., Flynn, H.A., Yoo, H., Marcus, S.M. & Davis, M.M. (2010). Risk Factors for Depressive Symptoms during Pregnancy: a Systematic Review. *Am J Obstet Gynecol,* Vol. 202, No. 1, (January 2010), pp. 5-14, ISSN 0002-9378

Levinson, D.J. (1996). *Seasons of a Woman's Life,* Alfred A. Knopf, ISBN 978-034-5311-74-0, New York, NY, USA

Llewellyn, A. M., Stowe, Z.N. & Nemeroff, C. B. (1997). Depression during Pregnancy and the Puerperium. *J Clin Psychiatry,* Vol. 58, Suppl, 15, pp. 26-32, ISSN 0160-6689

Luke, S., Salihu, H. M., Alio, A. P., Mbah, A. K., Jeffers, D., Berry, E. & Mishkit, V. R. (2009). Risk Factors for Major Antenatal Depression among Low-Income African American Women. *J of Women's Health,* Vol. 18, No. 11, (November 2009), pp. 1841-1846, ISSN 1540-9996

Morrison, D. F. (1990). *Multivariate Statistical Methods*, McGraw-Hill, ISBN 978-007-0431-87-4, New York, NY, USA

O'Hara, M. W. & Swain A. M. (1996). Rates and Risk of Postpartum Depression - a Meta-Analysis. *Int Rev Psychiatry*, Vol. 8, No. 1, (January 1996), pp. 37-54, ISSN 0954-0261

O'Hara, M. (1997). The Nature of Postpartum Depressive Disorders, In: *Postpartum Depression and Child Development*, L. Murray & P. J. Cooper (Eds.), pp. 3-31, The Guilford Press, 978-157-2301-97-9, New York, NY, USA

Peindl, K.S., Wisner, K.L. & Hanusa, B.H. (2004). Identifying Depression in the First Postpartum Year: Guidelines for Office-based Screening and Referral. *J Affect Disord, Disord*, Vol. 80, No. 1, (May 2004), pp. 37-44, ISSN 0165-0327

Pignone, M.P., Gaynes, B.N. & Rushton, J.L. & et al. (2002). Screening for Depression in Adults: a Summary of the Evidence for the U.S. Preventive Services Task Force. *Ann Intern Med*, Vol. 136, No. 10, (May 2002), pp. 765-776, ISSN 0003-4819

Plant, E. A. & Sachs-Ericsson, N. (2004). Racial and Ethnic Differences in Depression: the Roles of Social Support and Meeting Basic Needs. *J of Consulting and Clinical Psychology*, Vol. 72, No. 1, (February 2004), pp. 41-52, ISSN 0022-006X

Santrock J.W. (2008). *Life-Span Development*, McGraw-Hill Humanities Social, ISBN 978-007-3310-24-4, New York, NY, USA

Segre, L. S., O'Hara, M. W. & Losch, M. E. (2006). Race/Ethnicity and Perinatal Depressed Mood. *J of Reproductive & Infant Psychology*, Vol. 24, No. 2, (May 2006), pp. 99-106, ISSN 0264-6838

Segre, L. S., O'Hara, M. W., Arndt, S. & Scott Stuart. (2007). The Prevalence of Postpartum Depression: The Relative Significance of Three Social Status Indices. *Social Psychiatry and Psychiatric Epidemiology*, Vol. 42, No. 4, (April 2007), pp. 316-321, ISSN 0933-7954

Silverman, M. E., Loudon, H., Liu, X., Mauro, C., Leiter, G. & Goldstein, M. A. (2011). The Neural Processing of Negative Emotion Postpartum: a Preliminary Study of Amygdala Function in Postpartum Depression. Arch Women's Ment Health, Vol. 14, No. 4, (August 2011), pp. 355–359, ISSN 1434-1816

Surkan, P., Peterson, K., Hughes, M. & Gottlieb, B. (2006). The Role of Social Networks and Support in Postpartum Women's Depression: A Multiethnic Urban Sample. *Matern & Child Health J*, Vol. 10, No. 4, (July 2006), pp. 375-383, ISSN 1092-7875

Trevathan, W. (2010). *Ancient Bodies, Modern Lives: How Evolution Has Shaped Women's Health.* Oxford University Press, ISBN 978-019-5388-88-6, New York, NY, USA

Verinder, S., Vivien, K.B., & Hendrica, L.R. (2010). Assessment and Treatment of Bipolar II Postpartum Depression: A Review. *J Affective Disord.*, Vol. 125, No. 1, (September 2010), pp. 18-26, ISSN 0165-0327

Wei, G., Greaver, L.B., Marson, S.M., Herndon, C.H. & Rogers, J. (2008). Postpartum Depression: Racial Differences and Ethnic Disparities in a Tri-racial and Bi-ethnic Population. *Matern & Child Health J*, Vol. 12, No. 6, (November 2008), pp. 699-707, ISSN 1092-7875

Yonkers, K. A., Ramin, S. M., Rush, A. J. & et al. (2001). Onset and Persistence of Postpartum Depression in an Inner-city Maternal Health Clinic System. *Am J Psychiatry*, Vol. 158, No. 11, (November 2001), pp. 1856-63, ISSN 0002-953X

Zayas, L. H., Jankowski, K. B. & McKee, M. D. (2005). Parenting Competency Across Pregnancy and Postpartum Among Urban Minority Women. *J of Adult Development*, Vol. 12, No. 1, (January 2005), pp. 53-62, ISSN 1068-0667

# 9

# Postpartum Depression in Men

Sarah J. Breese McCoy
*Oklahoma State University Center for Health Sciences*
*Tulsa, Oklahoma*
*USA*

## 1. Introduction

Postpartum depression (PPD) is a form of major depressive disorder (MDD) and has traditionally been defined as occurring in women within three months to a year following childbirth (McCoy, 2011). However, this phenomenon has also been observed in men after their wives or partners give birth. The terminology used to described depression in males following the birth of a child has not yet been standardized. Some phrasing includes "paternal postpartum depression", and "postpartum psychiatric disorder, depressed mood, and distress" (Schumacher, 2008). For the purposes of this chapter, "paternal PPD" will be used. Although the research in men has been taking place for a much shorter time and with fewer patients than for women, valuable insights have already been gained.

## 2. Epidemiology and etiology

In any given year, about 3.3% of men experience general, true clinical depression, or MDD (Depression Facts and Statistics, 2009). Several attempts have been made to estimate the rate of paternal PPD, as well (Madsen & Juhl, 2007; Paulson & Bazemore, 2010; Lai, 2010). A meta-analysis of 43 studies from 16 countries estimated paternal PPD at 10.4%, with the highest rate occurring about 3-6 months postpartum (Paulson & Bazemore, 2010). That figure is suspiciously high, however, because the same analysis yielded an estimate of maternal PPD at 23.8%, well above the accepted average of 13% (Pearlstein et al, 2009; Cuijpers et al, 2008). These higher values are probably due to the inclusion of cases that may actually be only minor depression, without sufficient symptoms to qualify as MDD (Paulson & Bazemore, 2010). In fact, the true rate of paternal PPD may be closer to 5% (Madsen & Juhl, 2007). If paternal PPD were not a real phenomenon specifically related in some way to the birth of a child, the rate of men experiencing depression in the year following their children's birth would be expected not to exceed the 3.3% MDD incidence for men each year. In other words, any depression men might be experiencing in the postpartum period would be truly independent of and merely coincident with the child's birth.

Several factors have been shown to be independent predictors of paternal PPD: past history of severe depression, prenatal depression, prenatal anxiety, lower education level, having other children, and maternal prenatal depression (Ramchandani, 2008). Further, one finding in particular seems very clear—PPD in women influences paternal PPD. In fact, when maternal depression is moderate to severe, the prevalence of paternal PPD has been reported to be over 40% (Veskrna, 2010). In that same vein, the authors of the previously mentioned meta-analysis (Paulson & Bazemore, 2010) reached several useful conclusions: (1) Paternal PPD is a significant and real problem. (2) Rates are higher in the US than in other countries investigated, perhaps due to varying social norms or expectations. (3) Paternal PPD is correlated with maternal PPD.

Condon (2004) did a study at two teaching hospitals in Australia on 204 first-time fathers. Men were assessed using various mood and mental health scales at 23 weeks gestation, and at 3, 6, and 12 months after their partners gave birth. Interestingly, the fathers' greatest vulnerability to depression in the perinatal period was at the beginning of the third trimester of their partner's pregnancy, rather than after the birth. Although the authors admitted a possibility of sample bias, their results showed that expectant fathers were more likely to be depressed and irritable, had more somatic symptoms and even drank more alcohol than during the postpartum period. The reason for the fathers' stress and depression was apparently related to the anticipation of a decline in frequency of sex. Symptom measures were then relatively stable between 3 and 12 months postpartum. Another important finding was that during the first year postpartum, all significant relationship changes were in a negative direction between husband and wife, again, perhaps in large part from the men's point of view, because of decreasing frequency of sexual contact. Overall, however, the pregnancy itself was a more stressful time for men than the postnatal period (Condon et al, 2004).

## 3. Manifestations and consequences of male PPD

MDD in men and paternal PPD manifest somewhat differently than for women and may include such symptoms as hostility, conflict, and anger, rather than the more broadly recognized sadness or apathy (Table 1). In addition, men may self-medicate for their depression by drinking alcohol, and they may withdraw or engage in escape activities such as overwork, sports, sex, or gambling (Veskrna, 2010).

| | |
|---|---|
| 1. | Anger attacks |
| 2. | Affective rigidity (failure to express emotions) |
| 3. | Self criticism |
| 4. | Alcohol and drug abuse |
| 5. | Unhealthy sexual relationships or infidelity |
| 6. | Reckless behavior, such as unsafe driving |
| 7. | Abusive behavior |
| 8. | Escapist behavior, such as spending excessive time watching television or at work |

Table 1. Possible Additional Symptoms of Major Depressive Disorder in Men*
*www.mayoclinic.com; Madsen and Juhl, 2007

New fathers may experience many of the same changes and stresses that new mothers do, such as sleep disruption, relationship conflicts, and/or financial strain. Because many new mothers work, society now expects men to work more at home and help more with the children than in the past. Yet, their forbears, on whom those expectations did not rest, cannot provide an appropriate model for how to do this difficult task. The resultant stress may predispose men to a greater risk of depression in the postpartum period than at other times in their lives (Veskrna, 2010).

The literature has begun to suggest that fathers influence their children's attitude and actions more than was previously understood (Veskrna, 2010). For example, a United Kingdom study of 10,975 fathers and their children followed the families from 18 weeks gestation to seven years of age. This study was free of selection biases, and was prospective, which, together with its large sample size, were key strengths. Fathers were assessed four times—at 18 weeks gestation, eight weeks postpartum, eight months postpartum and twenty-one months postpartum. Their children were assessed at ages six and seven years, using reports from both the mothers and schoolteachers. The depression screens used for fathers in the study were the Edinburgh Postnatal Depression Scale (EPDS) and the Crown Crisp Experiential Index for anxiety symptoms (Ramchandani et al, 2008). The researchers found that paternal PPD at 8 weeks postpartum was associated with psychiatric diagnoses in their children at age seven years. In fact, twice as many children of depressed fathers developed a psychiatric disorder as children of fathers who were not depressed. Paternal PPD was also associated with higher scores on tests that measured sociability (reverse scored), hyperactivity, conduct problems, and peer problems. The authors concluded that paternal PPD is strongly predictive of increased rates of psychiatric disorders, such as oppositional defiant or conduct disorder, as well as social difficulties (Ramchandani et al, 2008).

In summary, adverse consequences to the child make paternal PPD especially important to address. New fathers should be evaluated for depression, especially when it is known that the mother is suffering from PPD. More research in this area is needed (Schumacher et al, 2008).

## 4. Making the diagnosis

As a form of MDD, PPD has traditionally been diagnosed according to the same criteria for MDD that are laid out in the Diagnostic and Statistical Manual-IV (DSM IV) (American Psychiatric Association, 2000) (Table 2). For a definitive diagnosis, five of the nine possible symptoms must be present for a minimum of two weeks. Instead of specific tests for PPD, sometimes regular screens for detecting MDD are used to assess women after they give birth. These include such tools as the Beck Depression Inventory (BDI), Center of Epidemiologic Studies Depression Scale (CES-D), and the Patient Health Questionnaire (PHQ-9), among others. Although the BDI is protected by copyright that prevents its demonstration here, the CES-D and the PHQ-9 are provided at the end of this chapter as a point of reference (Appendices 1 and 2).

Generalized tests are still used in PPD research, but they may give artificially elevated scores, because they count sleep disturbance and changes in appetite as symptoms of depression. However, both of these experiences are normal during the postpartum period, even for women who are not depressed (Pearlstein et al, 2009).

The Edinburgh Postnatal Depression Scale (EPDS) was developed as a screen specifically for PPD in women and first published in the literature in 1987. It is a self-administered, ten-question quiz in which participants rate how they have been feeling for the past week, selecting from four possible answers for each question. Each potential answer has a numerical value assigned to it, ranging from 0-3. The highest possible score on the test is 30, indicating the most depressive symptoms present. The lowest possible score is 0, indicating the least depressive symptoms (Appendix 3). The authors originally suggested that a positive screen for PPD be $\geq$ 13, for a demonstrated sensitivity and specificity of 86% and 78%, respectively (Cox et al, 1987). The EPDS is now well-established for use in both the prenatal and postpartum periods in women (Sit & Wisner, 2009) and has been translated into several languages.

| At least five of the following symptoms have been present during the same 2-week period; at least one of the symptoms is either #1 or #2 |
|---|
| 1. Depressed mood |
| 2. Diminished interest or pleasure in activities |
| 3. Significant change in weight or appetite |
| 4. Insomnia or hypersomnia |
| 5. Psychomotor agitation or retardation |
| 6. Fatigue or loss of energy |
| 7. Feelings of worthlessness or excessive or inappropriate guilt |
| 8. Diminished ability to think or concentrate |
| 9. Recurrent thoughts of death, suicidal ideation, suicide attempt or specific plan for committing suicide |

Table 2. Conventional Symptoms for Major Depressive Disorder in Men and Women*
*American Psychiatric Association, 2000

Investigation of the EPDS for use in men originated in the early 1990s. However, those first studies tended to use the same 12/13 cut-off for a positive screen as was recommended for English-speaking women. Women of some cultures now have lower cutoffs on the EPDS than English-speaking women, because they don't tend to be as demonstrative. In the same way, it makes sense that a positive screen for depression in men might be a lower score on the EPDS than for women, because men tend to express fewer negative emotions than women in Western cultures (Matthey et al, 2001).

The EPDS has two questions that deal with anxiety, and, therefore, it might also be used to detect fear and anxiety disorders as well as depression. Matthey et al (2001) uses the term "caseness" to refer to people who take the EPDS and meet the criteria for major/minor depression, or for panic, or adjustment disorder with anxiety. Matthey's study (2001) was done at 6-7 weeks postpartum, and 208 men participated. Of the 208, eleven met the criteria for distress—three with only depression, three with both depression and anxiety, and five with just anxiety. The optimum cutoff for men was 5/6, because with those values, 75% of distressed men and 69.8% of non-distressed men were correctly detected. False negatives were a mere 2.1%. Although the false positive rate was 87.3% at this cutoff, the authors felt it was justified, due to the great need to detect men with these disorders. The authors concluded that the EPDS is reliable and valid for detecting postpartum distress in men. They recommend that it be used routinely in all new fathers, as it has been recommend for use with all new mothers (Matthey et al, 2001).

In another investigation, 551 Chinese men were assessed with the EPDS and two other depression screens, the BDI and the Patient Health Questionnaire (PHQ-9), at eight weeks postpartum. The men's average age was about 33 years. The optimum cutoff score was set at ≥ 10, rather than ≥ 13 as recommended for English-speaking women. For a cutoff of 10/11, sensitivity was 91% and specificity was 97%. The EPDS was found to be more accurate than the other two screening tests. One reason seems to be that the EPDS does not include questions about fatigue and sleep disturbances as symptoms of depression, because they are both normal and common in new parents. Results showed that Chinese men were less likely than women to seek help for depression, but the rate of 3.1% of men meeting the criteria for depression was about the same as the rate for Australian fathers in another study. The symptoms most likely to be reported in both depressed and non-depressed fathers were feelings of being overwhelmed and blaming themselves unduly when things went wrong. The authors concluded that the postnatal period appears to be a time when Chinese men are vulnerable to developing depressive symptoms (Lai et al, 2010).

Because recent research is demonstrating that MDD in men, and thus paternal PPD, may manifest somewhat differently than depression in women, other screening tools that take into account men's unique symptoms are sometimes employed. One example is the Gotland Male Depression Scale (GMDS) (Table 3 & Appendix 4). Although it was not specifically designed for the postpartum period, its questions are engineered with the unique symptoms in mind of depression in males. Like the EPDS, the GMDS is self-administered and relatively easy to use. A cutoff score of > 13 is recommended as a positive result for depression. The GMDS has thirteen items and has been validated (Zierau et al, 2002).

| | |
|---|---|
| 1. | Lower stress threshold |
| 2. | Aggression, low impulse control |
| 3. | Feeling of being burned out or empty |
| 4. | Constant, inexplicable fatigue |
| 5. | Irritability, restlessness, dissatisfaction |
| 6. | Difficulty making decisions |
| 7. | Sleep problems |
| 8. | Anxiety/displeasure, especially in the morning |
| 9. | Abusive or hyperactive behavior; changes in eating habits |
| 10. | Antisocial behavior |
| 11. | Depressive thoughts |
| 12. | Increased tendency to complain |
| 13. | Family history of depression, alcoholism, suicide |

Table 3. Items Assessed in the Gotland Male Depression Scale (Madsen & Juhl, 2007)

A 2007 Danish study of 549 fathers calculated the prevalence of depressive symptoms at six weeks postpartum, using both the EPDS and the GMDS. Although neither test picked up all the fathers that were at risk for PPD, the EPDS was positive for 27 men, while the GMDS was only positive for eighteen (Madsen & Juhl, 2007). Ultimately, at this time there is no single ideal screening test for PPD in men, but the EPDS is probably the best tool available to date.

## 5. Treatment options

The standard of care for MDD in general continues to be antidepressants, psychotherapy, or both (McCoy, 2011). Paternal PPD is no exception. However, convincing men to seek help when they are depressed can be a challenge. Men are more likely to agree to psychotherapy if that option is presented as a way to protect or restore some aspect of their masculinity, as in the ability to provide for the family or contribute to the family's well-being (Veskrna, 2010).

Fletcher et al (2006) has listed some ideas for combatting paternal PPD that have already been tried with success in Australia or the United Kingdom. (1) Pamphlets for men about paternal PPD and the normal stresses and changes that accompany caring for a new baby can be sent home with new mothers when they visit an obstetrics clinic for a postpartum exam. (2) Prenatal classes can be offered that are specifically designed for men only and that are taught by male instructors. (3) A telephone help line may be designated for counseling fathers with questions or depressive symptoms (Fletcher et al, 2006).

A recent review article about PPD in women listed a few promising research areas for treatments in addition to the standard antidepressants and psychotherapy. Included were (1) managing sleep disturbances, such as minimizing exposure to light that disrupts the sleep cycle by using blue-blocking glasses when getting up to care for the infant in the night, (2) massage, and (3) exercise (McCoy, 2011). Although these options have not been researched in men, they are relatively inexpensive and safe and could make helpful additions to or in some cases, perhaps even alternatives to, traditional pharmaco- and psychotherapy.

## 6. Conclusions

Paternal PPD is a relatively new field of study, but it is established that the rate of depression in men during the postpartum period exceeds that for men in the population at large, probably somewhere between 3-5%. One important risk factor appears to be coincident PPD in the men's female partners, the new mothers. This disorder affects not only the men themselves, but also their children. In fact, the children of affected fathers may exhibit psychological disturbances and abnormalities even at the age of six or seven years. Although no perfect screening tool exists for detecting paternal PPD, the same EPDS that is used for women appears to be a valid instrument for screening men, particularly when a lower cutoff score is used. Treatments include antidepressants and psychotherapy and perhaps even some alternatives, but the main challenge at present is in convincing men that they need to seek help when they feel anxious, overwhelmed, angry, or sad. Educational and treatment programs that specifically target men experiencing PPD may make a significant contribution to the overall mental health of an entire family. Future research must focus on better education and public awareness about paternal PPD, better screening tools specifically for men, and treatment alternatives to psychotherapy or medications.

## 7. Appendix 1

**Center for Epidemiologic Studies Depression Scale (CES-D)**

Below is a list of some of the ways you may have felt or behaved. Please indicate how often you've felt this way during the past week. Respond to all items.

| Place a check mark in the appropriate column. | Rarely or none of the time (less than 1 day) | Some or a little of the time (1-2 days) | Occasionally or a moderate amount of time (3-4 days) | All of the time (5-7 days) |
|---|---|---|---|---|
| 1. I was bothered by things that usually don't bother me. | 0 | 1 | 2 | 3 |
| 2. I did not feel like eating; my appetite was poor. | 0 | 1 | 2 | 3 |
| 3. I felt that I could not shake off the blues even with help from my family. | 0 | 1 | 2 | 3 |
| 4. I felt that I was just as good as other people. | 3 | 2 | 1 | 0 |
| 5. I had trouble keeping my mind on what I was doing. | 0 | 1 | 2 | 3 |
| 6. I felt depressed. | 0 | 1 | 2 | 3 |
| 7. I felt that everything I did was an effort. | 0 | 1 | 2 | 3 |
| 8. I felt hopeful about the future. | 3 | 2 | 1 | 0 |
| 9. I thought my life had been a failure. | 0 | 1 | 2 | 3 |
| 10. I felt fearful. | 0 | 1 | 2 | 3 |
| 11. My sleep was restless. | 0 | 1 | 2 | 3 |
| 12. I was happy. | 3 | 2 | 1 | 0 |
| 13. I talked less than usual. | 0 | 1 | 2 | 3 |

| Place a check mark in the appropriate column. | Rarely or none of the time (less than 1 day) | Some or a little of the time (1-2 days) | Occasionally or a moderate amount of time (3-4 days) | All of the time (5-7 days) |
|---|---|---|---|---|
| 14. I felt lonely. | 0 | 1 | 2 | 3 |
| 15. People were unfriendly. | 0 | 1 | 2 | 3 |
| 16. I enjoyed life. | 3 | 2 | 1 | 0 |
| 17. I had crying spells. | 0 | 1 | 2 | 3 |
| 18. I felt sad. | 0 | 1 | 2 | 3 |
| 19. I felt that people disliked me. | 0 | 1 | 2 | 3 |
| 20. I could not "get going." | 0 | 1 | 2 | 3 |

Source: Radloff, LS (1977). The CES-D scale: A self-report depression scale for research in the general population. Applied Psychological Measurement, 1:385-401.

Directions: Do not score if missing more than 4 responses. (1) For each item, look up your response and corresponding score (0-3). (2) Fill in the score for each item under the last column labeled "Score." (3) Calculate your Total Score by adding up all 20 scores.

Scoring Results: Total Score of 16 or higher is considered depressed. If your score indicates depression, see a health care/mental health professional for further evaluation and treatment. Bring these test results to your appointment.

## 8. Appendix 2

**Patient Health Questionnaire-9**

Over the last 2 weeks, how often have you been bothered by any of the following problems?

| Use a check mark to indicate your answer. | Not at all | Several days | More than half the days | Nearly every day |
|---|---|---|---|---|
| 1. Little interest or pleasure in doing things. | 0 | 1 | 2 | 3 |
| 2. Feeling down, depressed, or hopeless | 0 | 1 | 2 | 3 |
| 3. Trouble falling or staying asleep, or sleeping too much | 0 | 1 | 2 | 3 |

| Use a check mark to indicate your answer. | Not at all | Several days | More than half the days | Nearly every day |
|---|---|---|---|---|
| 4. Feeling tired or having little energy | 0 | 1 | 2 | 3 |
| 5. Poor appetite or overeating | 0 | 1 | 2 | 3 |
| 6. Feeling bad about yourself – or that you are a failure or have let yourself or your family down | 0 | 1 | 2 | 3 |
| 7. Trouble concentrating on things, such as reading the newspaper or watching television | 0 | 1 | 2 | 3 |
| 8. Moving or speaking so slowly that other people could have noticed? Or the opposite – being so fidgety or restless that you have been moving around a lot more than usual | 0 | 1 | 2 | 3 |
| 9. Thoughts that you would be better off dead or of hurting yourself in some way | 0 | 1 | 2 | 3 |

**FOR OFFICE CODING** 0 + ______ + ______ + ______
**= Total Score:** ______

Developed by Drs. Robert L. Spitzer, Janet B.W. Williams, Kurt Kroenke and colleagues, with an educational grant from Pfizer Inc. No permission required to reproduce, translate, display or distribute.

## 9. Appendix 3

**Edinburgh Postnatal Depression Scale**

How Are You Feeling?

As you have recently had a baby, we would like to know how you are feeling now. Please underline the answer which comes closest to how you have felt in the past 7 days, not just how you feel today.

Here is an example, already completed:

I have felt happy:

- Yes, most of the time
- <u>Yes, some of the time</u>
- No, not very often
- No, not at all

This would mean: "I have felt happy some of the time" during the past week. Please complete the other questions in the same way.

IN THE PAST SEVEN DAYS

1. I have been able to laugh and see the funny side of things:
   - As much as I always could
   - Not quite so much now
   - Definitely not so much now
   - Not at all
2. I have looked forward with enjoyment to things:
   - As much as I ever did
   - Rather less than I used to
   - Definitely less than I used to
   - Hardly at all

*3. I have blamed myself unnecessarily when things went wrong:
   - Yes, most of the time
   - Yes, some of the time
   - Not very often
   - No, never

4. I have felt worried and anxious for no very good reason:
   - No, not at all
   - Hardly ever
   - Yes, sometimes
   - Yes, very often

*5. I have felt scared or panicky for no very good reason:
   - Yes, quite a lot
   - Yes, sometimes
   - No, not much
   - No, not at all

*6. Things have been getting on top of me:
   - Yes, most of the time I haven't been able to cope at all

- Yes, sometimes I haven't been coping as well as usual
- No, most of the time I have coped quite well
- No, I have been coping as well as ever

*7. I have been so unhappy that I have had difficulty sleeping:
- Yes, most of the time
- Yes, sometimes
- Not very often
- No, not at all

*8. I have felt sad or miserable:
- Yes, most of the time
- Yes, quite often
- Not very often
- No, not at all

*9. I have been so unhappy that I have been crying:
- Yes, most of the time
- Yes, quite often
- Only occasionally
- No, never

*10. The thought of harming myself has occurred to me:
- Yes, quite often
- Sometimes
- Hardly ever
- Never

Response categories are scored 0, 1, 2, and 3 according to increased severity of the symptom. Items marked with an asterisk are reverse scored (i.e. 3, 2, 1 and 0). The total score is calculated by adding together the scores for each of the ten items. Users may reproduce the scale without further permission providing they respect copyright (which remains with the *British Journal of Psychiatry*) by quoting the names of the authors, the title and the source of the paper in all reproduced copies.

## 10. Appendix 4

**The Gotland Scale for assessing male depression**

Wolfgang Rutz, MD, PhD, Psychiatrist, Visby
Zoltan Rihmer, MD, PhD, Psychiatrist, Budapest
Arne Dalteg, PhD, Psychologist, Visby
English version: Per Bech, Lis Raabaek Olsen, Vibeke Norholm, Psykiatrisk Forskningsenhed, Hillerod

During the past month, have you or others noticed that your behavior has changed, and if so, in which way?

| | **Not at all** | **To some extent** | **Very true** | **Extremely so** |
|---|---|---|---|---|
| 1. Lower stress threshold/more stressed out than usual | 0 | 1 | 2 | 3 |

| | Not at all | To some extent | Very true | Extremely so |
|---|---|---|---|---|
| 2. More aggressive, outward-reacting, difficulties keeping self-control | 0 | 1 | 2 | 3 |
| 3. Feeling of being burned out and empty | 0 | 1 | 2 | 3 |
| 4. Constant, inexplicable tiredness | 0 | 1 | 2 | 3 |
| 5. More irritable, restless and frustrated | 0 | 1 | 2 | 3 |
| 6. Difficulty amking ordinary everyday decision | 0 | 1 | 2 | 3 |
| 7. Sleep problems: sleeping too much/too little/restlessly, difficulty falling asleep/waking up early | 0 | 1 | 2 | 3 |
| 8. In the morning especially, having a feeling of disquiet/anxiety/uneasiness | 0 | 1 | 2 | 3 |
| 9. Overconsumption of alcohol and pills in order to achieve a calming and relaxing effect. Being hyperactive or blowing off steam by working hard and restlessly, jogging or other exercises, under- or overeating | 0 | 1 | 2 | 3 |
| 10. Do you feel your behavior has altered in such a way that neither you yourself nor others can recognize you, and that you are difficult to deal with? | 0 | 1 | 2 | 3 |
| 11. Have you felt or have others perceived you as being gloomy, negative or characterized by a state of hopelessness in which everything looks bleak? | 0 | 1 | 2 | 3 |
| 12. Have you or others noticed that you have a greater tendency to self-pity, to be complaining or to seem "pathetic"? | 0 | 1 | 2 | 3 |

| | Not at all | To some extent | Very true | Extremely so |
|---|---|---|---|---|
| 13. In your biological family, is there any tendency toward abuse, depression/dejection, suicide attempts or proneness to behavior involving danger? | 0 | 1 | 2 | 3 |

Total Score: ________
0-13: No signs of depression.
13-26: Depression possible. Specific therapy, including psychopharmacological, possibly indicated.
26-39: Clear signs of depression. Specific therapy, including psychopharmacological, clearly indicated.

## 11. References

American Psychiatric Association. Diagnostic and Statistical Manual of Mental Disorders, Fourth Edition, Text Revision. Washington, DC: American Psychiatric Association, 2000.

Condon JT, Boyce P, Corkindale CJ. (2004). The First-Time Fathers Study: a prospective study of the mental health and wellbeing of men during the transition to parenthood. Aust N Z J Psychiatry 38:56-64.

Cox JL, Holden JM, Sagovsky R. (1987). Detection of postnatal depression. Development of the 10-item Edinburgh Postnatal Depression Scale. Br J Psychiatry 150:782-786.

Cuijpers P. (2008). Psychological treatment of postpartum depression: a meta-analysis. J Clin Psychol 64:103-18.

Depression Facts and Statistics. (2009) "Clinical Depression" http://www.depressionperception.com/depression/depression_facts_and_statistics.asp#clinical (Accessed August 16, 2011).

Fletcher RJ, Matthey S, Marley CG. (2006). Addressing depression and anxiety among new fathers. MJA 185(8):461-3.

Lai BP, Tang AKI, Lee DTS, Yip ASK, Chung TKH. (2010). Detecting postnatal depression in Chinese men: a comparison of three instruments. Psychiatry Res 180(2-3): 80-5.

Madsen SA, Juhl T. (2007). Paternal depression in the postnatal period assessed with traditional and male depression scales. JMHG 4(1):26-31.

Male Depression: Understanding the Issues. www.mayoclinic.com/health/male-depression/MC00041. Accessed August 10, 2011.

Matthey S, Barnett B, Kavanagh DJ, Howie P. (2001). Validation of the Edinburgh Postnatal Depression Scale for men and comparison of item endorsement with their partners. J Affect Disord 64:175-184.

McCoy SJB. (2001). Postpartum depression: An essential overview for the practitioner. Southern Med J 104(2):128-132.

Paulson JF, Bazemore SD. (2010). Prenatal and postpartum depression in fathers and its association with maternal depression: a meta-analysis. JAMA 303(19):1961-9.

Pearlstein T, Howard M, Salisbury A, Zlotnick C. Postpartum depression. (2009) Am J Obstet Gynecol 200:357-64.

Radloff, LS. (1977). The CES-D scale: A self-report depression scale for research in the general population. Applied Psychological Measurement 1:385-401.

Ramchandani PG, Stein A, O'Connor TG, Heron J, Murray L, Evans J. (2008). Depression in Men in the Postnatal Period and Later Child Psychopathology: A Population Cohort Study. J Am Acad Child Adolesc Psychiatry 47(4):390-398.

Schumacher M, Zubaran C, White G. (2008). Bringing birth-related paternal depression to the fore. Women Birth 21(2): 65-70.

Sit DKY, Wisner KL. (2009). Identification of postpartum depression. Clin Obstet Gynecol. 52:456-68.

Veskrna, L. (2010). Peripartum depression - does it occur in fathers and does it matter? JMH 7(4):420-430.

Zierau, F., Bille, A., Rutz, W., & Bech, P. (2002). The Gotland male depression scale: A validity study in patients with alcohol use disorder. *Nordic Journal of Psychiatry,* 56, 265-271.

# 10

# Risk Factors of Postnatal Depression Among Immigrants in Norway

Soen Eng Yap and Babill Stray-Pedersen
*Women and Childrens's Division, Oslo University Hospital, Rikshospitalet and Institute of Clinical Medicine, University of Oslo, Norway*

## 1. Introduction

### 1.1 Migration

Migration is not a new phenomenon, it has become an integral and inevitable part of global and economic development. Better communication and easier and faster transport system increases both voluntary and forced migration. The United States, Canada, and Australia were built on migration, and most European countries were saved by being able to send millions of people to other places when confronted with massive agricultural, political, or economic crises. Illness and death rates associated with migration are exacerbated by a lack of policies needed to make migration a healthy and socially productive process. Migrants are typically poor people moving from poor economic environments, they carry with them the health profiles that result from poverty. Migrants can also be healthy people with initiatives and economy to migrate. Migration, even under the best of conditions, involves a series of events that can be highly traumatizing and that can place migrants at risk. From a public health point of view, migration has serious ramifications for the people that move, the family they leave behind, and the communities that host the newcomers. Migration means breaking with family, friends, and established social networks, departing from traditional routines, value system, feeling of isolation, and these all are often detrimental to both mental health and social integration (Carballo M 2001).

Migration is a process of social change whereby an individaul moves from one cultural setting to another for the purpose of settling down in the new environment either permanently or for a prolonged period (Syed HR 2003). Migration is a complex and dynamic process that can impact the health of migrants, both positively and negatively depending on a number of conditions associated with invidual, social, environmental and health related factors. Immigrant health has therefore been regarded as a public health challenge in several countries (Abebe DS 2010).

Migration is often associated with major changes in environment and behavior, most notably changes in dietary habits, nutrient intake and physical activity influenced by a process of urbanization or westernization. This has subsequently led to an increased risk of chronic diet- and lifestyle-related diseases in ethnic minority groups (Misra A 2007, Gilbert PA 2008). Several studies over the past decades have indicated an increased risk of obesity, diabetes, CVDs and Vitamin D deficiency in immigrant communities as compared to their country of origin and the mainstream population (Abebe DS 2010).

Before 1960s, Norway was a homogeneous country. Thereafter, a considerable migratory influx of economic immigrants, particularly from Pakistan, Morocco and Turkey, has occurred. After restriction for working purposes was imposed in 1975, immigration has been limited to refugees, asylum seekers, special labors, family reunion and marriages. The first Pakistani men came to Norway as economic immigrants 40 years ago. Most women came for marriage, and most were cousins or relatives of their husbands. In Oslo, the capital of Norway, 28 % of the population are immigrants or Norwegian-born to immigrant parents where the Pakistani comprises the largest immigrant group (13%) (Statistics Norway 2011).

Psychological health may be affected by the process of leaving family and coping with job insecurity, legal problems, unfamiliar language and culture. Stress and anxiety can result in more serious psychological problems (Liebkind 1996). Psychological distress is a measure of mental health, represented by symptoms of anxiety, depression and somatization. The ethnic Pakistanis reported a higher prevalence of psychological distress 22.0% as opposed to 9.9% in ethnic Norwegians (Syed HR 2006). Furthermore, the Oslo Health Study found that the prevalence of psychological distress among immigrants from low- and middle-income countries was signicicantly higher than among the immigrants from high-income countries. Both pre- and post-migration factors were associated with distress. However, the post-migration factors were the most important indicators for the difference between the two groups of immigrants. Lack of salaried job, recent negative life events, past traumatic experiences, living without a partner, low social support, poor knowledge of Norwegian language were associated with mental distress (Hauff E 2006).

To-day there has been a growing interest in acquiring a better understanding of the health status and healthcare needs of our immigrants.

## 2. Postnatal depression

Women are at an increased risk for first onset of major depression from early adolescence until their mid-50s and have a lifetime rate of major depression 1.7 to 2.7 times greater than that of men. Risk of depression increases in some periods of a woman's life and the postnatal period is one of these (Burt VK 2002). Mental diseases are frequent and among the most common complications associated with women's pregnancies and childbirth (Brockington I 2004). Unipolar depression is the most common type, but bipolar affected illness, obsessional disorders and anxiety may also occur and represent a considerable health problem that affects not only the women but also their children and family ( Brockington I 2004, Sinclair D 1998).

There are three postpartum psychiatric disorders - the maternity blues, puerperal psychosis and postnatal depression (Brockington I 2004). Postpartum psychosis is generally defined as any mental disorder occurring within three months after childbirth and serious enough to require admission to psychiatric facility (David HP 1981). Childbirth, together with abortion (David HP 1981) and menstruation (Brockington I 2005), are those of the triggers of bipolar episodes in susceptible women.

Postnatal depression generally occurs within 6-8 weeks after childbirth (Patel V 2002). It is a significant public health problem with a prevalence varying from 4.9 to 28 % (Bjerke SEY 2008, Chandran M 2002, Rahman A 2003, Ho-yen SD 2006) with the highest value reported from Chile (50.7%) (Poo F AM 2008). While a meta-analysis has shown an average prevalence of 13 % in the general population (O'hara MW 1996).

The Pakistani immigrants represent a minority group with a very different culture compared with Norwegians, and they may feel very alienated from their Norwegian counterparts (Bjerke SEY 2008). In addition, rates of prenatal and postnatal depression in Pakistan has been reported as high as 28% to 41% (Rahman A 2003, Muneer A 2009, Khooharo Y 2010) .Thus, we might expect higher prevalence of depression in this group compared with ethnic Norwegians.

## 3. Reproductive health among immigrants

Reproductive health especially among women seems to be affected by changes in social and economic environment, nutritional and lifestyle transition, access to education and health care. Pregnancy-related illnesses and pregnancy problems among migrants are common throughout Europe (Carballo M 2001).

The changing of society from traditional agricultural to increasingly urban industrial is known to be followed by a demographic transition from high to low fertility. Women's education and work force participation are suggested as key predictors of the fertility transition (Caldwell J 1999, Bongaarts J 2003).

Total fertility rate in Norway is 1.95, among the highest in Europe, only Iceland and Ireland have higher fertility rate than Norway (Statistics Norway 2011). In 1990, total fertility rate among Pakistani immigrants was 4, nowadays a little more than 3. Second generation Pakistani immigrants has almost the same rate as Norwegians, those which came as children have higher fertility rates that is clearly declining, and lower than women who immigrated as adults (Statistics Norway 2010). In general, immigrants from Asia, Africa and Latin-America have higher rates than the ethnic Norwegian population (Statistics Norway 2010).

We still have a limited knowledge of the migration and health of women of reproductive years, although our knowledge of migration and health is increasing.

In Norway, mean birth weights have been low for Vietnamese and Pakistan mothers and high for Norwegian and North African mothers (Vangen S 2002). In the United Kingdom, perinatal and postnatal mortality are higher among immigrants born in Pakistan and Caribbean than the general population (Carballo M 2001).

Unwanted pregnancies, poor knowledge about familyplanning and where to get contraceptive devices and advice are common among immigrant women. Request for abortion tend to be higher among immigrants from Africa and South America than Spanish women (Carballo M 2001). A study in Italy reported the risk of induced abortion being higher among the foreigners (34.8/1000 women) than among the residents (10.5/1000 women). However, the spontaneous abortion ratio was also higher among the foreigners (213.8/1000 live births) than the residents (154.6/1000 live birthes) (Medda E 2002).

In Norway immigrant women from Asia and Africa seem to experience a higher risk of obstetric-related complications, perinatal mortalities and higher rates for the termination of pregnancies in comparison to Norwegians and Western immigrants (Abebe DS 2010). The risk factors were female genital mutilaton, consanguineous marriages, low or inconsistent use of contraception, low education and poor socioeconomic status. In addition, a lack of experience and knowledgse among health workers and communication problems between healthcare providers and immigrant patients were mentioned as possible challenges ( Abebe DS 2010).

To-day, childbirths are significantly more common among Pakistani women than among Norwegians in Oslo. Report suggests that low education is associated with high frequencies of induced abortion among Norwegians, while Pakistani women with higher education on the contrary are more likely to undergo induced abortion (Eskild A 2007). Overall, non-Western immigrant women seem to represent a risk group for induced abortion in Norway (Eskild A 2002), especially refugees and labour migrants had significantly higher termination of pregnancy (TOP) rates than nonmigrants. NorwayTOP rate was 16.7 per 1000 women contra Pakistani 18.4 (Vangen S 2008).

## 4. Risk factors of postnatal depression

Past history of psychological disorder (Bjerke SEY 2008, O'hara MW 1996), psychological disorder during pregnancy, low socioeconomic status, complicated delivery (O'hara MW 1996), high scores on the life event scale and poor marital relationship were reported as risk factors of postnatal depression (Bjerke SEY 2008, Eberhard-Gran M 2002). Feeling anxious during pregnancy has been a strong predictor of inctrasing symptoms of depression within 6-8 weeks after birth. However, university education and friends's support appear to be important protective factors (Grussu P 2009). Public postnatal care lowered the risk of postnatal depression (McArthur 2002). Early discharge from the maternity wards (Hickey AR 1997) , young age (Inandi T 2002, Irfan N 2003), being single (Bjerke SEY 208, Kendell RE 1987), high parity (Danaci AE 2002), low education and illeteracy (Inandi T 2002, Irfan N 2003), birth of a daughter when a son was desired (Chandran M 2002, Patel V 2002), lack of physical help (Chandran M 2008), as well as being an immigrant (Danaci AE 2002, Small R 2003) have also been reported as risk factors for postnatal depression.

## 5. Material and methods

### 5.1 Study population and method

The Pakistani immigrants are the largest immigrant group in Oslo, Norway. We wanted to investigate this immigrant group in order to better understand of our new fellow citizens. The recruitment were performed when the Pakistani women came for prenatal ultrasound screening in 17-18 gestational week at two maternity hospitals in Oslo (Rikshospitalet and Ullevål University Hospitals). Women from the two regions in Oslo (Grunerløkka and Grønland) where most of the Pakistani women lived were randomly included. Although we had asked the midwifes and their assistants to assemble the Pakistani women on one particular day when the author was able to visit, it happened quite often that none or only one patient was registered, and thus home visits were necessary. After two years, we had included 207 women. Every one of them gave their personal consents and signatures.

Two face-to-face interviews: one prenatal and one 6-12 weeks after delivery were performed. Ten women did not have the postnatal interview. These included one woman who suffered from a late miscarriage, two women with stillbirths, and one whose baby died a few days after delivery. Three women had moved to Pakistan, one woman refused to be interviewed, one to an unknown address and one woman had been killed. This left a total of 197 women that were interviewed twice. Almost half of the participants (91 women) did speak and understood Norwegian. For the remaining, professional interpreters were used or family members were acting as interpreters.

The questionnaire employed after birth was designed as a structured questionnaire ( Eberhard-Gran M 2002) which included EPDS, in order to access the prevalence of and risk factors of postnatal depression.

The Edinburgh Postnatal Depression Scale (EPDS) is a 10-item self-rating scale designed to identify post-natal depression (Cox JL 1987). The EPDS has been translated into Norwegian and validated (Eberhard-Gran M 2001). EPDS items concern matters such as having been able to laugh, having looked forward with enjoyment to things, having blamed oneself unnecessarily, having been anxious or worried for no good reason, having felt scared or panicky for no good reason, experiencing overload, having been so unhappy that it has caused sleeping problems, having felt miserable or sad, having so unhappy as to have cried, thoughts of harming oneself. Each EPDS item is scored 0-3 and the maximum total score is 30.

We aimed at including all Pakistani women registered for ultralsound prenatal screening at two hospitals in the study. Most women in the Oslo area are giving birth at these hospitals. Thus we believe that selection bias in the sample is minimal.

The study was approved by the Regional Committee for Ethics and Research and the Data Inspectorate.

### 5.2 Variables

The structure questionnaire included collection of the following information: *Demographic and socioeconomic factors.* Age, marital status, relationship, family structure, educational level, parity, family income, employment status, years of residence in Norway. *Reproductive factors and history.* Mean age of menstrual debut and premenstrual debut and premenstrual complaints, the number of children, previous miscarriages, previous induced abortions, stillbirths and pregnancy complications such as hyperemesis gravidarum, pelvic pain, pregnancy experience, length of time to become pregnant without contraception, mode and length of delivery, person(s) present at delivery, anxiety and mood during labour, contentment with hospital stay, breastfeeding, the sex and health of the baby. *Somatic diseases.* Incidence during the previous year, information obtained by answering the following checklist: asthma, hay fever/allergy, high-blood pressure, cardiovascular disease, diabetes, thyroid disease, gynecological disease, muscular/skeletal/articular disease, migraine/headache, cancer or other somatic diseases not listed above. *Psychiatric history.* History of hereditary depression, previous depression. *Interpersonal relationship.* The participant has persons outside the family that she can confide in that, helps her with housework, or care for the family. The coding is 'yes' or 'no'. Attachment to partner was asked for and codes as 'closely attached to partner', 'partly' or 'not attached at all'.

*Life events.* Major life events during the last 12 months. The live events included 10 different items:1) separation or divorce; (2) serious problems in marriage or cohabitation; (3) problems or conflict with family, friends or neighbors; (4) problems at work or in place of education; (5) economic problems; (6) serious illness or injury; (7) serious illness or injury within the nuclear family/among close family members; (8) traffic accident, fire or theft, (9) loss of a closely related persons; and (10) other difficulties. The answers were graded according to the woman's reaction to the event; not so difficult/difficult/very difficult, and the sum of scores from each item (graded according to severity on a scale of 1-3) was used as a negative life event indicator (codes:'0 points', '1-5 points', or '>5 points'). The women with 0 points reported 0 major events.

*Outcome variable. Measures of mental health.* EPDS was included in the questionnaire. The EPDS scores were dichotomized in the statistical analyses as high score (≥10) or low score (<10) (Eberhard-Gran M 2002).

### 5.3 Statistical analyses

All data were registered in SPSS. Descriptive statistics (including means, standard deviations, frequencies and percentage) were used to analyze distribution of the demographic variables.

Crude odds ratios for being depressed (EPDS≥10) with 95% confidence intervals were estimated by logistic regression analyses.

**The aims** of our study was to investigate the risk factors for postnatal depression among immigrant women especially Pakistani living in Norway.

## 6. Results

A total of 197 Pakistani women completed the study; 15 (7.6%) suffered from postnatal depression as seen in Table 1 (EPDS score ≥10) (Bjerke SEY 2008). The average age of our study was 28.0 years ( range 19-43 years; SD 5.0. The majority (97%) were married and more than one-third lived in extended families, 70% had more than one child.

None of the Pakistani women had a university level education, 67 (34%) had a high school level, 54 (27%) had only 9 years of schooling, while one was illiterate. Most of the women (69%) were unemployed (Table 1).

The different risk factors and their significance for postnatal depression are given in Tables 1 and 2 (Bjerke YSE 2008).

Advanced age was one risk factor: 14% of the 79 women over 30 years old suffered from postnatal depression. This was significantly different from the 3 % depression rate observed in the 118 women under 30 years (OR 4.6, 95% Cl 1.4-15.0).

Among the five mothers who for different reasons were single, three women were depressed after delivery (OR 22.5, 95% Cl 7.1-124.1).

Considering the women with prior depression, six out of 10 suffered from a new episode of depression in the postnatal period (OR 29.7, 95% Cl 7.1-124,1).

Of the 12 women who were not closely attached to their partners, four (33%) suffered from postnatal depression (OR 8.6, 95% Cl 2.2-33.5).

Out of the total 197 women, 26 (15%) women scored high on the life-event scale. Half of these suffered from postnatal depression with a high OR (84.5, 95% Cl 17.2-415.2).

In fact 13 of the 15 (87%) of those experiencing postnatal depression had previously had a distressing lift event.

| | EPDS > 10 | | | |
|---|---|---|---|---|
| Risk factor | Yes, *N* (%) | No, *N* (%) | Total *N* | Crude odds-ratio (95% CI) |
| | 15 (7.6) | 182 (92.4) | 197 | |
| Age of the woman | | | | |
| < 30 years | 4 (3) | 114 (97) | 118 | 1 |
| > 30 years | 11 (14) | 68 (86) | 79 | 4.6 (1.4–15.0)* |
| Marital status | | | | |
| Married | 12 (6) | 180 (94) | 192 | 1 |
| Single | 3 (60) | 2 (40) | 5 | 22.5 (3.4–147.8)* |
| Family structure | | | | |
| Nuclear | 9 (7) | 121 (93) | 130 | 1 |
| Extended | 6 (9) | 61 (91) | 67 | 1.3 (0.5–3.9) |
| Unemployment | | | | |
| No | 2 (3) | 59 (97) | 61 | 1 |
| Yes | 13 (10) | 123 (90) | 136 | 3.1 (0.7–14.3) |
| Educational level | | | | |
| 9 years of school | 3 (6) | 51 (94) | 54 | 0.8 (0.2–3.7) |
| High school level | 7 (10) | 60 (90) | 67 | 1.7 (0.5–5.5) |
| University level | 0 (0) | 0 (0) | 0 | 0 |
| Others | 5 (7) | 71 (93) | 76 | 1 |
| Number of children | | | | |
| > 1 child | 13 (9) | 125 (91) | 138 | 1 |
| 1 child | 2 (3) | 57 (97) | 59 | 3.0 (0.6–13.6) |

*Statistical significance.

Table 1. Relative risk of postpartum depression expressed as odds ratios with a 95% confidence interval according to demographic and socio- economic factors among 197 Pakistani Women.

| Risk factor | EPDS ≥ 10 Yes, N (%) | No, N (%) | Total | Crude odds-ratio (95%CI) |
|---|---|---|---|---|
| | 15 (7.6) | 182 (92.4) | 197 | |
| Premenstrual tension | | | | |
| No | 2 (3) | 66 (97) | 68 | 1 |
| Slight | 11 (10) | 99 (90) | 110 | 3.7 (0.8–17.1) |
| Noticeable – annoying | 2 (11) | 17 (89) | 19 | 3.9 (0.5–29.6) |
| History of spontaneous abortion | | | | |
| No | 11 (7) | 153 (93) | 164 | 1 |
| Yes | 4 (12) | 29 (88) | 33 | 1.9 (0.6–6.4) |
| History of stillbirth | | | | |
| No | 13 (7) | 176 (93) | 189 | 1 |
| Yes | 2 (25) | 6 (75) | 8 | 4.5 (0.8–24.6) |
| Mode of last delivery | | | | |
| Vaginal delivery without complications | 9 (6) | 146 (94) | 155 | 1 |
| Vaginal delivery with strain | 2 (12) | 15 (88) | 17 | 2.2 (0.4–11) |
| Operative delivery | 4 (16) | 21 (84) | 25 | 3.1 (0.9–11) |
| Breastfeeding | | | | |
| No | 2 (25) | 6 (75) | 8 | 1 |
| Yes | 13 (7) | 176 (93) | 189 | 0.2 (0.4–12) |
| Somatic diseases | | | | |
| No | 14 (9) | 145 (91) | 159 | 1 |
| Yes | 1 (3) | 37 (97) | 38 | 0.3 (0.0–2.2) |
| Prior depression | | | | |
| No | 9 (5) | 178 (95) | 187 | 1 |
| Yes | 6 (60) | 4 (40) | 10 | 29.7 (7.1–124.1)* |
| Interpersonal relationship | | | | |
| Yes | 13 (7) | 174 (93) | 187 | 1 |
| No | 2 (20) | 8 (80) | 10 | 0.3 (0.6–1.6) |
| Closely attached to partner | 10 (6) | 172 (94) | 182 | 1 |
| Partly or not attached to partner | 4 (33) | 8 (67) | 12 | 8.6 (2.2–33.5)* |
| No partner | | 3 | | |
| Life events | | | | |
| 0 point | 2 (1) | 169 (99) | 171 | 1 |
| More than one point | 13 (50) | 13 (50) | 26 | 84.5 (17.2–415.2)* |

*Statistical significance.

Table 2. Relative risk of postpartum depression expressed as odds ratio with a 95% confidence interval according to sociological and biological factors among 197 Pakistani women.

## 7. Discussion

We found that the prevalence of postnatal depression (EPDS score ≥10) among Pakistani women in Norway was only 7.6%, slightly lower than that of the ethnic Norwegian (8.9%) (Eberhard-Gran M 2002), and lower than reported elsewhere in the world (13%) ( O'Hara MW 1996). Depression around childbirth is a serious public health problem in south Asia, affecting about one in four women (Patel V 2002). In Pakistan prevalence of postnatal depression were reported up to 41% (Rahman A 2003, Muneer A 2009, Khooharo Y 2010). The prolonged maternal depression has various consequences not only for the mother but also for infant growth and development (Rahman A 2007).

Many previous studies have shown risk factors for postnatal depression similar to those we have revealed in this study.

The interview was performed in Norwegian, not in 'Urdu', the original Pakistani language. Half of our women spoke Norwegian, while for the remaining, professional interpreter and family members were used as interpreters. The presence of family members during the interview might have led to underreporting of depressive symptoms (Cox JL 1987). However, we analyzed the results of those 'to be alone' and those 'who had their husband with them' and found no significant difference of depressive symptoms. The EPDS is based on self- rating. This implies that the women should be able to read, understand, and cross off correspondingly. For an illiterate person, this is not possible. In an interview situation there could also be a risk of under-reporting psychiatric symptoms (Ho-Yen SD 2006). In Nigeria, reading out psychometric questionnaires to illeterate people did not alter the psychometric properties of the instrumens used (Abiodun OA 1994). Kirmayer showed that disturbances in mood, effect and anxiety are not viewed as mental health problems in many cultures, but rather of a social or moral nature (Kirmayer LJ 2001). It is possible that immigrant Pakistani women did not perceive depression as a mental problem (Bjerke YSE 2008).

In an ethnic Norwegian study, the risk factors were beeing primiparous, not having breastfed, having a prior depression, poor attachment to partner and high stress of life-event ( Eberhard-Gran M 2002). Our Pakistani immigrants had some of the similar risk factors to ethnic Norwegian: prior depression, poor attachment to partner and high stress of life-event.

Current somatic illness (Chandran M 2002, Small R 2003) and life stress have been reported to be important risk factors for postnatal depression (Eberhard-Gran M 2002). This is in accordance with our results, which showed that a high score on life events was strongly associated with the depressed condition. Almost everyone, 13 out of 15 with postpartum depression had previously suffered from a traumatic lift event. The same risk factor was registered in Pakistan (Rahman A 2007).

Previous psychiatric illness (Eberhard-Gran M 2002, Irfan N 2003, Ho-Yen SD 2007), depression during pregnancy were reported as risk factors for postnatal depression (Rahman A 2007, Ho-Yen SD 2007). In our study all women with prior depression, suffered of postnatal depression. Previous postnatal depression is also considered a risk factor in Pakistan (Khooharo Y 2010).

Being single is a wellknown risk factor (Kendell RE 1987). From a traditional and cultural standpoint, being a single mother is even worse and considered to be a shame in Asia. We confirmed this risk factor even thorught we had only three of five women in our study in this category (Bjerke SEY 2008). This is in contrast to Norway where being a single mother no longer is a burden (Eberhard-Gran M 2002).

Social isolation and poor relationships with their spouses and the spouse's parents have been shown to be risk factors for postnatal depression (Chandran M 2002, Danaci AE 2002, Lee DT 2004). In a British study, Pakistani mothers living in extended families were more depressed and anxious than those in nuclear families (Shah Q 1995). Perhaps Pakistani women in Norway did not feel socially isolated, because one-third lived in extended families and none of these reported depression, in contrast to Pakistani women in their origin country, who reported postnatal depression (Muneer A 2009, Khooharo Y 2010). However, because the majority of husbands were present at the interview, the reliability of our data in this respect is questionable. However, poor attachment was the risk factor in our study and ethnic Norwegian study (Eberhard-Gran M 2002, Bjerke SEY 2008) , also in Pakistan (Khooharo Y 2010).

Previous reproductive failure or problems such as stillbirth have been related to depression and anxiety in the next pregnancy and puerperium (Hughes PM 1999). Among our Pakistani women, two suffered from stillbirth in the current pregnancy, but they were excluded from the postnatal questionnaire. When considering a history of previous stillbirths, eight women (4%) had experienced these events, 25% of these women were depressed. However, the results were not significant, because our study was not large enough to study such rare events.

Women who experience stress during childbirth (Watson JP 1984, O'hara MW 1996), or emergency delivery have been shown to have an incidence of twice the risk of developing postnatal depression (Koo V 2003). We had 42 women (21%) in this category, but only six (14%) suffered from postnatal depression and we thus did not confirm this risk factor.

Breastfeeding did not influence postnatal depression in our study. This is in contrast to the study by Alder where mothers exclusively breastfed their babies for at least 12 weeks, or who were taking contraceptives, had a higher incidence of postnatal depression than those who were not 'on the pill' or who partially breastfed (Alder EM 1983). Postnatal depression has been shown to have a significant negative impact on breastfeeding duration in other studies (Misri S 1997).

The risk of postnatal depression was in previous studies mainly related to socio economic and family variables (Chandran M 2002): young age (Inandi T 2002, Irfan N 2003), high parity (Danaci AE 2002, Ho-Yen SD 2007), the gender of the child (female) (Chandran M 2002), low education and illiteracy (Inandi T 2002, Irfan N 2003), financial difficulties and low social class (Inandi T 2002, Irfan N 2003), being a housewife (Inandi T 2002, Irfan N 2003), being an immigrant (Danaci AE 2002, Small R 2003). These factors did not show an association to postpartum depression among Pakistani women in our study. However, in Pakistan: young age (Muneer A 2009, Khooharo Y 2010), low level of education (Muneer A 2009, Khooharo Y 2010), lower socioeconomic class (Muneer A 2009, Khooharo Y 2010. Rahman A 2007), small families comprising of fewer than 3 children (Muneer A 2009), having 5 or more children (Rahman A 2007), lack of a confidant or friend (Rahman A 2007), were married for less than 5 years (Muneer A 2009), domestic violence (Khooharo Y 2010) and house wives (Khooharo Y 2010) were reported as risk factors.

Integration is a question of equal rights in society, which is a central part of Norwegian immigration policy: In 1997, the Norwegian government declared that immigrants should have the same rights to health care as the rest of the population (Ministry of Local and Labor 1997). Integration is also a question of equity in health outcomes. This may explain that in Norway being an immigrant or belonging to different socio-economic groups do not give different health outcomes compared with ethnic Norwegians (Eberhard-Gran M 2002) and Pakistani women in the rural districts of Pakistan (Rahman A 2007).

Limitation of the study should be discussed, since the author only once a week was coming to Oslo for interviewing the immigrants, and probably not recruited all wanted women.

**In conclusion,** the 7.6% prevalence of postnatal depression among Pakistani women in Norway seems to be very low compared with the prevalence reported in immigrant populations elsewhere, however it was only slightly lower than the ethnic Norwegians (8.9%).

Being a Pakistani immigrant in Norway does not seem to result in a higher risk of postnatal depression. The different risk factors are similar to those reported from other countries; moreover, the there seemed to be few cultural differences in risk factors between the ethnic Norwegian and Pakistani immigrants.

In the future the role of the immigrant father should be further looked into. Prenatal and postnatal depression occurring in the fathers has been described in up to 10% (Paulson J 2010), with a relatively higher frequency in the 3- to 6- month postnatal period. Paternal depression has showed a moderate correlation with maternal depression (Paulson J 2010). This is interesting and future studies should focus upon postnatal depression in males and their risk factors.

## 8. References

Abiodun DA. A validity study of the Hospital Anxiety and Depression Scale in General Hospitals units and a community sample in Nigeria. Br J Psychiatry 1994; 163:670-672.

Abebe DS. Public Health Challenges of immigrants in Norway: A Research Review. NAKMI report 2/2010.

Alder EM, Cox JL. Breast feeding and post-natal depression. J Psychosom Res. 1983;27:139-144.

Bjerke SEY, Vangen S, Nordhagen R, Ytterdahl T, Magnus P, Stray-Pedersen B. Postpartum depression among Pakistani women in Norway: prevalence and risk factors. J Matern Fetal Neonatal Med2008;21:889-894.

Bongaarts J. Completing the fertility transition in the developing world: The role of educational differences and fertility preferences. Popul Stud 2003;57:321-336.

Brockington I. Postpartum psychiatric disorders. Lancet 2004;363:303-310.

Brockington I. Menstrual psychosis. World Psychiatry 2005;4:9-17.

Burt VK, Stein K. Epidemiology of depression throughout the female life cycle. J Clin Psychiatry 2003;63:9-15.

Caldwell J. Paths to lower fertility. BMJ 1999;319:985-987.

Carballo M, Nerukar A. Migration, Refugees, and Health Risks. Emerging infect. Dis.2001;7:556-560.

Chandran M, Tharyan P, Muliyil J, Abraham S. Post-partum depression in a cohort of women from a rural area of Tamil Nadu, India. Incidence and risk factors. Br. J Psychiatry 2002;181:499-504.

Cox JL, Holden JM, Sagovsky R. Detection of postnatal depression. Development of the 10-item Edinburgh Postnatal Depression Scale. Br J Psychiatry 1987;150:782-786.

Danaci AE, Dinc G, Deveci A, Sen FS, Icelli I. Postnatal depression in Turkey: epidemiological and cultural aspects. Soc Psychiatr Epidemiol 2002; 37:125-129.

David HP, Rasmussen NK, Holst E. Postpartum and postabortion psychotic reactions. Fam Plann Perspect 1981;13:88-89.

Eberhard-Gran M, Eskild A, Tambs K, Schei B, Opjordsmoen S. The Edinburgh postnatal depression scale: Validation in a Norwegian community sample. Nord J Psychiatry 2001;55:113-117.

Eberhard-Gran M, Eskild A, Tambs K, Samuelsen S, Opjordsmoen S. Depression in postpartum and non-postpartum women: prevalence and risk factors. Acta Psychiatr Scand 2002;106:426-433.

Eskild A, Helgadottir LB, Jerve F, Qvigstad E, Stray-Pedersen S, Løset A. Induced abortion among women with foreign cultural background in Oslo ( in Norwegian). Tidsskr Nor Lægeforen. 2002;122:1355-1357.

Eskild A, Nesheim BJ, Busund B, Vatten L, Vangen S. Childbearing or induced abortion: the impact of education and ethnic background. Population study of Norwegian and Pakistani women in Oslo, Norway. Acta Obstet Gynecol Scand.2007:86:298-303.

Gilbert PA, Khokhar S. Changing dietary habits of ethnic groups in Europe and implications for health. Nutr Rev 2008;66:203-215.

Grussu P, Quatraro RM. Prevalence and risk factors for a high level of postnatal depression symptomatology in Italian women: a sample drawn from antenatal classes. Eur Psychiatry 2009;24:327-333.

Hauff E. The mental health of immigrants: recent findings from the Oslo Health study 2006.

Hickey AR, Boyce PM, Ellwood D, Morris-Yates AD. Early discharge and risk for postnatal depression. Med J Aust 1997;167:244-247.

Ho-Yen SD , Bondevik GT, Eberhard-Gran M, Bjorvatn B. The prevalence of depressive symptoms in the postnatal period in Lalitpur district, Nepal. Acta Obstet Gynecol Scand 2006;85:1186-1192.

Hughes PM, Turton P, Evans CD. Stillbirth as risk factor for depression and anxiety in the subsequent pregnancy: Cohort study. BMJ 1999;318:1721-1724.

Inandi T, Elci OC, Ozturk A, Egri M, Polat A, Sahin TK. Risk factors for depression in postnatal first year, in eastern Turkey. Int J Epidemiol 2002;31:1201-1207.

Irfan N, Badar A. Determinants and pattern of postpartum psychological disorders in Hazara division of Pakistan. J Ayub Med Coll Abbottabad 2003;15:19-23.

Kendell RE, Chalmers JC, Platz C. Epidemiology of puerperal psychoses. Br J Psychiatry 1987;150:662-673.

Khooharo Y, Majeed T, Das C, Majeed N, Choudhry AM. Associated risk factors for postpartum depression presenting at a teaching hospital. ANNALS 2010;16:87-90.

Kirmayer LJ. Cultural variations in the clinical presentation of depression and anxiety: Implications for diagnosis and treatment. J Clin Psychiatry 2001;62:22-28.

Koo V, Lynch J, Cooper S. Risk of postnatal depression after emergency delivery. J Obstet Gynaecol Res 2003;29:246-250.

Lee DT, Yip AS, Leung TY, Chung TK. Ethnoepidemiology of postnatal depression. Prospectice multivariate study of sociocultural risk factors in a Chinese population in Hong Kong. Br J Psychiatry 2004;184:34-40.

Liebkind K. Acculturation and stress: Vietnamese refugees in Finland. Journal of Cross-Cultural Psychology 1996;27:161-180.

McArthur C, Winter H, Bick DE, Knowles H, Lilford R, Henderson C et al. Effects of redesigned community postnatal care on womens' health 4 months after birth: a cluster randomised controlled trial. Lancet 2002;359:378-385.

Medda E, Baglio G, Guasticchi G, Spinelli A. Reproductive health of immigrant women in the Lazio region of Italy. Ann Ist Super Sanita 2002:38:357-365.

Ministry of Local Government and Labour. Immigration and the multicultural Norway ( in Norwegian). St.meld.nr.17, 1997.

Misra A. Ganda OP. Migration and its impact on adiposity and type 2 diabetes. Nutrition 2007;23:696-708.

Misri S, Sinclair DA, Kuan AJ. Breast-feeding and postpartum depression: Is there a relationship? Can J Psychiatry 1997;42:1061-1065.

Muneer A, Minhas FA, Tamiz-ud-Din Nizami A, Mujeeb F, Usmani AT. Frequency and associated factors for postnatal depression. J Coll Physicians Surg Pak. 2009;19:236-239.

O'hara MW, Swain AM. Rates and risk of postpartum depression-a meta-analysis. Int rev Psychiatry 1996;8:37-54.

Paulson, JF, Bazemore SD. Prenatal and postpartum depression in fathers and its association with maternal depression. A meta-analysis. JAMA 2010;303:1961-1969.

Patel V, Rodrigues M, DeSouza N. Gender, poverty and postnatal depression: a study of mothers in Goa, India. Am J Psychiatry 2002;159:43-47.

Poo F AM, Espejo SC, Godoy PC, Gualda de la CM, Hernandez OT, Perez HC. Prevalence and risk factors associated with postpartum depression in puerperal women consulting in primary care. Rev Med Chil.2008;136:44-52.

Rahman A, Iqbal Z, Harrington R. Life events, social support and depression in childbirth: perspectives from a rural community in the developing world. Psychol Med 2003;33:1161-1167.

Rahman A, Creed F. Outcome of prenatal depression and risk factors associated with persistence in the first postnatal year: Prospective study from Rawalpindi, Pakistan. J. Affect Disord.2007;100:115-121.

Shah Q, Sonuga-Barke E. Family structure and the mental health of Pakistani Muslim mothers and their children living in Britain. Br J Clin Psychol 1995;34:79-81.

Sinclair D, Murray L. Effects of postnatal depression on children's adjustment to school. Teachers's reports. Br J Psychiatry 1998;172:58-63.

Small R, Lumley J, Yelland J. Cross-cultural experiences of maternal depression: Associations and contributing factors for Vietnamese, Turkish and Filipino immigrant women in Victoria, Australia. Ethn Health 2003;8:189-206.

Statistics Norway. Population statistics, immigrant population, 2009. Available: http://no.wikipedia.org/wiki/Pakistanere i Norge.

Statistics Norway. Population statistics, immigrant population, 2010. Available: http://www.ssb.no/befolkning/main.shtml

Statistics Norway. Population statistics, immigrant population, 2011. Available: http://www.ssb.no/befolkning/main.shtml

Syed HR, Vangen S. Health and migration: a review. National Center for Minority Health Research and National Institute of Public Health;2003. Report No.:2.

Syed HR, Dalgard OS, Hussain A, Dalen I, Claussen B and Ahlberg NL. Inequalities in health: a comparative study between ethnic Norwegians and Pakistanis in Oslo, Norway. Int J Equity Health 2006;5:7.

Vangen S, Stoltenberg C, Skjærven R, Magnus P, Harris JR, Stray-Pedersen B. The heavier the better? Birthweight and perinatal mortality in different ethnic groups. Int J Epidemiol 2002;31:654-660.

Vangen S, Eskild A. Forsen L. Terminationof pregnancy according to immigration status: a population-based registry linkage study. BJOG 2008;115:1309-1315.

Watson JP, Elliot SA, Rugg AJ, Brough DI. Psychiatric disorder in pregnancy and the first postnatal year. Br J Psychiatry 1984; 144:453-462.